Praise for EcoChi: Designing the Human Experience

"Debra Duneier has taken the art of sustainable interior design to its next logical level. The world would be a better place if everyone read this book and followed her guidelines."

—John Messerschmidt, Vice President of Operations, Green City Challenge

"In this ground-breaking new book, Debra Duneier transforms how we live and work. The EcoChi system builds a better world, one person at a time, and enhances the quality of our lives and the success of our businesses. This book will inspire you to discover how to align who you are with a world that is designed to support your life and your work."

—Sharon Emek, Vice President, Women's Builders Council
President/CEO of Work at Home Vintage Employees LLC.

"Debra Duneier has combined her credentials in all aspects of interior design—from environmental to spiritual—to flesh out what we need to know and do with our surroundings to insure a successful, joyous life. The future will be about experience, and the personal experience of our living and working spaces is central to that future. I know people who have been profoundly transformed by Debra's work. EcoChi is a must read!"

—Edie Weiner, President, Weiner, Edrich, Brown, Inc.

"In this delightful new book, Debra Duneier helps to transform how we live and work and, in the process, build a better world, one person and one building at a time."

—Susan Stautberg, Co-Founder/Co-Chair, WomenCorporateDirectors (WCD)
President, PartnerCom

"Debra Duneier makes complex issues easy to understand, and she offers such telling and delightful anecdotes not only about designing spaces but also about designing our lives. EcoChi was so much fun to read and it moved me into action immediately. Since implementing several of Debra's suggestions, I feel the energy shifting positively already!"

—*Leslie Grossman, Co-Founder, Women's Leadership Exchange*
Author, SELLsation!

"EcoChi: Designing the Human Experience is an absolute "must read" if you want to enhance your life by gaining control over your personal living and work space. Congratulations, Debra, on helping us to improve our lives with your insight and sage advice."

—*Susan Solovic, CEO/Co-Founder/Owner, SBTV.com*

"Debra Duneier writes a useful, thought-provoking book on bringing humanity into the spaces we inhabit—our homes and our offices—making sure they are spiritual as well as environmentally sound."

—*Shirley Moulton, Founder, The ACADEMi of Life*

"Debra Duneier shares her strategies for transforming our indoor spaces by bringing nature indoors. If you read only one book on renovation or design this year, it should be EcoChi: Designing the Human Experience. It's brilliant!"

—*Nicole Hollant-Denis, President, AARRIS Architects*

"Debra has successfully blended the ancient wisdom of classical feng shui with modern concepts of green and sustainable living and environmental psychology. EcoChi presents practical solutions that are easy to implement. This is a sure key to success in business and in life!"

—*Alan Ceppos, Co-Chairman/Co-Founder, Pylones USA*

EcoChi

DESIGNING THE HUMAN EXPERIENCE

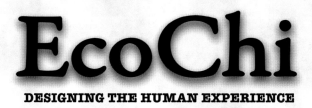

BY DEBRA DUNEIER

New Voices Press
New York, New York

New Voices Press
315 West 70th Street
New York, NY 10023
212-580-8833

An application to register this book for cataloguing
has been submitted to
the Library of Congress.

ISBN 978-0-9748103-8-6
1. Architecture - Decorative arts 2. Fine Arts - Decoration
and decorative furnishings 3. Ecology - Human ecology -
Environmental influences on humans 4. Social Sciences -
Life skills 5. Philosophy – Chinese – Feng Shui
6. Technology - Home economics - the house

Book design by Bruce Jacobson

Dedicated to my children Danielle Duneier-Goldberg
and Jamie Troy Duneier, who are an infinite source of
inspiration, joy and light in my life.
My love for you cannot be expressed sufficiently in the
written word; it can only be read on my soul.

Life is lived the way it is designed ...

Contents

Acknowledgements

It is with deep gratitude and respect that I take this moment to thank all of the people who have touched my life profoundly with their knowledge, talents, inspiration and love. You have taught me that each of us has the power to positively impact others, as you have influenced my life with your light and presence.

My journey has been a beautiful unfolding because of the teachers who generously shared their wisdom with me along the way. Some are professors, scientists and masters. Others are clients, friends, neighbors and loved ones. All have contributed to my life, my heart, my spirit and my work and I am grateful.

I would like to express my deep appreciation, to Master Nan Lu, who advised me to pursue my gift, and to the teachers that followed: Roger Green, Nam Singh, Janus Welton, Patricia Michael, Jean Haner, Marnie Muller, Mark Hanf, Michael Rice, Kristen Bacorn, Ester Muller, Joan Mahon, E.J Shaffert and the teachers at the Holis Institute.

To all of my "sisters": thank you for your friendship, encouragement and unwavering confidence in me and my work. I treasure you, Edie Weiner—you are an eternal source of love and support in my life. Goldie Forman, your love of music, song and dance lives on in EcoChi. Forever in my heart, I am thankful for the time we shared together here on Earth.

Every author understands that a book editor is an invaluable component to their finished product. Thank you, Judy Katz and Bonnie Egan.

To my artistic team, I am in admiration of your talents and tenacity; Jeremy Mack, book cover and EcoChi logo design; Bruce Jacobson, book design; Holden Jay, Photography; Susan Kroll, Stylist; Selenia Perez, Make-up and hair.

I would like to give special recognition to my son Jamie Duneier, a television writer by profession, for his notes, late night conversations and always reminding me above all to trust my inner voice.

Lastly, I would like to express my profound appreciation to Robert Friedland, my partner in life and in love, for his encouragement, patience and his unparalleled faith in me and my work. My life is complete and full with him by my side, and it is with great excitement that I look ahead, as we continue to explore life and its endless possibilities together.

Introduction

Every space has a life of its own, and impacts us as we go about our lives. Our actions, energy and thoughts, as well as our physical well-being, are all profoundly influenced by our surroundings. The design, color scheme, textures, light, furnishings, accessories and placement of each item in our indoor environments impact our senses from moment to moment and shape how we feel about ourselves and others. This is true whether we are at home, at work or in public spaces such as hotels, spas, hospitals, conference centers, retail stores and office buildings. This heightened understanding of how our interiors affect us both consciously and unconsciously is the solid foundation of the EcoChi System—the system I created and now implement in both residential and commercial properties.

EcoChi is more than design. It's a lifestyle shift that meticulously blends the powerful ancient and modern lessons of classical feng shui, green and sustainable living and environmental psychology to revolutionize how people feel when they are inside a building. Most of us spend 99% of our time indoors. When we are at work at our desks, watching sports on television, eating our meals at home or in restaurants, playing video games or enjoying museums or theater, it is easy to forget our connection to the outdoor world. Still, some of the happiest moments of our lives are spent outdoors. We all have recollections of these experiences—a blazing sunset, the scent of the ocean air, animal life encountered on a stroll through the woods, the view of a pastel sunrise from a mountaintop, a golden harvest moon or the fleeting glimpse of a mammoth butterfly.

In Eastern philosophy, it is believed that life and the natural world are inseparable from one another. As we become more attentive to nature, we become more aware of ourselves. During my studies, I realized that if I could find ways to bring nature's elements into indoor spaces, the effects on the inhabitants would be extremely positive. The possibilities of benefits seemed innumerable:

- Attainment of personal goals such as wealth, love, happiness
- Physical and mental well-being
- Moving forward after a loss or crisis
- Taking back the reins of control over one's life
- Living in harmony and balance

When applied to businesses, it also adds other organic benefits:

- Improving ROI (Return on Investment)
- Happier employees resulting in lower turnover
- Healthier working environment and reduced absenteeism
- Satisfied customers and brand loyalty
- Environmental responsibility for our planet and lower energy costs

Introduction

Once I realized the potential of EcoChi, my passion deepened. The idea of sharing this with as many people as possible became my life's work.

What is unique about EcoChi? How do I combine these disciplines in a way that offers transformational results? I will answer these questions in the chapters ahead and share with you how EcoChi performs in my own life, in businesses, public spaces and the lives of individuals. Many people generously shared their stories about their personal and business experiences with me. To protect their confidentiality, I have changed their names and other identifying characteristics. But their stories are true, and the results were, if anything, even more remarkable than I can adequately convey.

By implementing the EcoChi system, you can open doors to new possibilities that will advance you professionally, while also bringing greater joy to you in all aspects of your personal life. EcoChi favorably impacts not only the inhabitants of a space, but also those who visit, work in spaces you provide or spend leisure time in public spaces you create. As you are about to discover, EcoChi is truly an equal opportunity transformational system.

My world was falling apart. The foundation under my feet felt like it was crumbling. Everything I worked for and depended on was no longer in place. I felt I was in free fall...

The Birth of EcoChi

The birthing of EcoChi was a happy accident, one that began, as many such life-changing journeys often do, with a confluence of overwhelming events. One such event was the dot-com crash, which just about wiped out the Internet-based corporate gift business I had built and run with great success over the previous 17 years. Days filled with hundreds of orders became days when there were almost none. My business was in critical condition, so I was forced to close the larger of my two factories and reduce payroll by letting go of nonessential employees and cutting hours back for others. I also canceled any back orders with my suppliers. Debra Hope Creations, Inc. was on life support.

On September 11th, 2001, the terrorist attacks on the World Trade Center and the Pentagon took our loved ones before their time, rocked our souls and left our emotions raw. It was also devastating to businesses. This event landed the second knockout punch to my company and it was down for the count.

It was during that time that I went to Chinatown to visit a Chinese Master of Acupuncture that a friend had recommended. I had a frozen shoulder and it was very painful. My doctor had me on a variety of anti-inflammatory drugs and excruciating physical therapies. Nothing was working but I was determined to avoid surgery. My friend Donna suggested that I give alternative medicine a try. I have to be honest with you; the thought of having a complete stranger sticking needles in my body made me queasy. This was also my first trip into Chinatown so the whole experience was very foreign, and I was definitely out of my comfort zone. As I lay on the table, the Master tried to move my arm over my head. It would not budge. The first thing he asked me was "Where are you stuck in your life?"

Where *wasn't* I stuck? My business had just taken its last breath, but that was only part of the story. After a marriage of 25 years, I was in the middle of a painful divorce, one I did not want and had not seen coming. My son was away at college and my daughter was about to leave for her first semester at George Washington University. I was going to be stuck in a 5,000-square-foot house, coping with empty nest syndrome, in a suburban town where I had never felt I belonged. My only companion was Bradley, an angry standard poodle, who also missed having the family around him. I was no longer a wife, no longer had my children home and was no longer president of my own company. Where was I stuck? Everywhere!

Gently and with great skill the Master strategically placed the needles into my skin. It felt strange, like a pinch, but it was not as painful as I anticipated. I could feel a wave of energy moving around the needles and all over my body, inside and out. Suddenly, the Master broke the silence: "You have a gift." I held my breath, hoping he would say more. What was he talking about? After a few moments had passed, he added this: "Do not waste it." That said, he walked out of the room and closed the door behind him.

Stunned by his words, I lay there, reflecting on my life, and on what in the world my "gift" could be.

Overwhelmed by "Stuff"

I had married my high school sweetheart just three days after my 19th birthday. We built a highly successful jewelry manufacturing business together and had enjoyed, for the vast majority of that time, what was truly a close family life. Now, with my husband and children gone, the packing up of all our lives was left to me. Of course, I was overwhelmed—not just emotionally but also on a practical level by all of the "stuff" my family had accumulated in the twenty years we'd been in our comfortable, spacious home. I knew much of it would have to go, but making those decisions seemed monumental. I could not possibly fit all my things and all my children's things into a much smaller city apartment. I would have to make strategic decisions, or take too much with me and live in a cluttered environment.

I have never liked clutter, but one thing I had yet to learn in a more conscious way was how accurately the state of your surroundings reflects the state of your life. If your home or office is filled with clutter, there is no room for new and wonderful things to come into your life or career. Clear out the spaces and you shift the energy. What's wonderful is that you can often feel the difference almost immediately. In my case I started the process of de-cluttering with baby steps, one drawer and then one closet at a time. The Chinese Master had challenged me to find out where I was stuck in my life so I could let it go and move on. I decided I would try. I felt like I had nothing left to lose. I didn't even know who I was anymore. His words were powerful and I hung on to them as if they were my lifeline. Still, at that moment, I felt rudderless, lost at sea, devastated.

Determined to attack my clutter in a methodical manner, I created what I call "The SMG System" (Stay, Maybe and Go). I shopped for containers of various sizes. Then I began to work my way through all my possessions. Anything I hadn't used in a year went into the "Go" pile except for the things that I still found it difficult to separate from. Those went into the "Maybe" pile. The things I was still using went into the "Stay" containers, which I clearly labeled with permanent markers. Over the next few weeks I dumped, donated and packed.

What surprised me was how many things started to easily flow from the "Maybe" to the "Go" pile. If it was a sentimental item that evoked a memory but was definitely not something I would have room for in my new place, I found that if I took a photo of it I could more easily let it go. The longer I looked at various items—clothing, furniture, letters, and so much more that I had accumulated in my daily life—the more I realized that, in truth, I did not need them. With this new attitude, the all-important "Go" pile kept growing.

I had to make a very difficult decision about the family dog. Based on my love for him and understanding of his needs, I knew that Bradley would never be happy in a small apartment in Manhattan. I found a family that lived right on Virginia Beach who fell in love with Bradley and were thrilled to adopt him. Suddenly, with lots of room to run and play and a new household full of love, Bradley was no longer angry. In fact, this wonderful animal brought great joy to this family, whose young mother was fighting cancer. So he too found a second life. Happily, a lot of what I gave away has brought a measure of pleasure to others. This was the beginning of my deeply gratifying and exciting new work—helping others realize their dreams by bringing beauty and harmony to their interiors and into their lives.

Making Room for a New Future

An unexpected and ultimately priceless benefit of this entire meltdown, and the reflective process it forced on me, was that I learned who I really was. Cutting ties, material and otherwise, allowed me to explore the world in a new way. The path I was now following was, for the first time in my life, my own path—not anyone else's. I had gotten my divorce, sold my house, moved into an apartment in Manhattan and closed my business. My next move was to study for my broker's license and begin a new career in high-end residential sales. At first, all went beautifully and sales were brisk. But in 2007 the housing bubble burst. The ensuing global financial meltdown hit everyone very hard and my business was no different. My sales quickly dropped by about 30 percent and continued to plummet. So much for the longevity of my new career as a real estate broker!

A New Topic Galvanizes an Audience

In the midst of all this I was invited to speak at an international business conference. The organizers asked me to make a list of possible subjects for my presentation. I sent in about 20 topics, including: "How to create your real estate team"; "How to choose your real estate attorney"; "How to prepare your property for sale"; and "Feng Shui." I actually had some knowledge about feng shui but, to this day, I am not sure why I put it on the list. As fate would have it, that was the topic they chose, so I had to do some research and become more familiar with the subject before the presentation.

I gave my talk. Afterwards, a line of people formed, all wanting to speak with me one-on-one about some aspect of feng shui. Something had shifted inside me and something extraordinary was happening. As I spoke briefly with each person on that line, I felt an intense personal connection with each individual. The topic was clearly one of great importance to them, and when I had my moment with each one, it was like there was no one else in the room.

Returning home from this successful presentation, I discovered nothing but escalating bad news about the real estate market. If I was going to reinvent myself, I would have to act fast and be resilient. As a problem solver and one who generally tries to look on the bright side of things, I viewed this state of affairs as an opportunity. Thinking back on the unexpected and overwhelming reception to my presentation, I decided to study with a Feng Shui Master to learn more about this fascinating discipline and see where it would take me. As it happens, the person I chose was one of three Feng Shui Masters who were credited with bringing feng shui to the U.S. from China in the 1960s. As I studied with him, expanding my knowledge of the art and science of indoor and outdoor spaces, I kept in mind that unusual jolt of connectivity I had felt with each person at that conference who had asked me about feng shui. Something wonderful was definitely happening inside of me and it was bubbling up to the surface.

We all have gifts but sometimes it takes the right circumstances or the right person at the right time to lead you to them. Fortunately the Chinese Master appeared at the precise time in my life when I was ready to let go of my past and embrace my new path. It actually took me seven years to find my gift. It was a process of self-discovery, combined with extensive and intensive study of both the ancient and the modern. Most of all, it required being open to whatever the universe had in mind for me.

Interestingly, at this moment in time, I feel like I am standing on a key "acupuncture point" in the universe and a turning point in our earth's history. My hope, in creating EcoChi, is that it has the power and possibility, if utilized by each of us and enough of us, to serve as one of the "needles" that can bring back the vital resurgence of positive energy we so urgently need in our spaces... and in our lives.

In the pages ahead I will share my journey of discovery and disclose the endless opportunities available to you when living the EcoChi experience.

The Birth of EcoChi

ECOCHI IS BUILT ON THE

FUNDAMENTAL BELIEF THAT

"HOME" IS WHEREVER YOU

ARE, AND THAT IT IS

ESSENTIAL TO NURTURE YOUR

INDOOR SPACE SO THAT IT

NURTURES THE SPIRIT

WITHIN.

Chapter Two

A Recipe for Transformation Takes Shape

Kitchens inspire me. While I love every room that makes up a home, I must admit that I find kitchens especially enchanting. This is the heart of the home, a place where love can be expressed through creativity. In fact, I have never lost my sense of awe at how one can take a classic recipe, and with a pinch of this and a dash of that, something delicious and original is born. Given my adventurousness in the kitchen, it is exhilarating and not really surprising to me that all the hard work and the years of accumulating knowledge in a variety of disciplines has led me to the creation of the new discipline I call EcoChi. EcoChi is built on a solid foundation of three basic, tried and true ingredients: feng shui, green and sustainable living, and environmental psychology.

I will soon describe all three prongs of this discipline in detail. EcoChi has given me what I wanted so badly for so long: a powerful strategy to help people experience their spaces in an entirely new way, and in so doing, transform their lives.

A Whole Greater Than the Sum of Its Parts

In the early 80s, I looked for and found every entrepreneur's dream, an unmet niche in the marketplace, and I established Debra Hope Creations, Inc. This online gift service was designed specifically to provide businesses and organizations with the type of gift item they could be proud of sending out for corporate events and special occasions. The custom-designed gift baskets I created were received with raves, reorders and referral business. Like most endeavors of passion, creating these packages was, for me, the highest form of self-indulgence.

The process itself was so much fun. I would choose a basket from my inventory—anything from a painted basket with handles to a natural wood tray. Working out of my design studio, I would blast Rod Stewart on the stereo and begin the creative process while singing, dancing and sipping a freshly brewed cup of decaf hazelnut coffee. First, I would place an array of products into this basket, which acted as the "pot." This could include gourmet foods, chocolates, bath products, stationary and other items of all shapes, sizes, colors, scents and tastes. These were my "ingredients." I would then design my end product, which was something magnificent and far beyond its individual components. My "recipe" was then entered into the computer, with the list of components and a photograph so each design could be exactly reproduced for future orders.

The music I listened to, the colors and scents with which I surrounded myself, the taste of hazelnut and the panoply of textures I worked with all brought joy to my life because they engaged all of my senses and created a wonderful Chi energy. As a result, Debra Hope Creations became a successful international business with happy employees and delighted customers. I tell you this story because forming and running that company lives on in EcoChi— the pinnacle of all my many lessons learned. So here are the basic ingredients, which, once imbued with my own "secret sauce," became the **EcoChi System**.

Feng Shui

Feng shui is a design method that involves purposefully arranging a space so that it has an uplifting and life-enhancing effect on the people who occupy that environment. When designing beautiful buildings, rooms and outdoor spaces, it takes into consideration the surrounding aspects of nature and the specific landscape and topography of a site.

The ancient Chinese, undistracted by television, cell phones and the Internet, devoted their time to studying the mysteries of life. They masterfully created fundamental disciplines and life-enhancing applications, all based on their strong appreciation and understanding of the natural world. Lying on their backs at night and looking up at the stars, these Chinese sages studied the universe, nature's cycles and the relationships these cycles created. They then translated these relationships into numbers and symbols (Trigrams). This is how feng shui was born.

Feng shui literally means "wind and water" in Cantonese. Wind represents the shifting energies (Chi). Water represents contained Chi at rest. Chi (qi) is the dynamic movement of non-tangible energy or vibrations. In India it is known as *prana,* in Japan *ki,* in Arab nations *Baraka,* and for Polynesians *mana.* In the western world we have no word to express this concept. The closest description in our language is "life force." With feng shui, one can enhance and amplify the Sheng Chi (auspicious energy) and eliminate or minimize the Sha Chi (inauspicious energy) in order to bring about a desirable balance.

Many people with little or no knowledge of feng shui think of it as merely moving furniture around to reposition it in some more advantageous location. That is so not the case! Having studied feng shui for years, I can tell you that there are no shortcuts to understanding all aspects of this intuitive art. Feng shui, like an onion, has many layers. The most well known School of Classical Feng Shui is called Form School. Form School consultants work with Earth Chi—the forms of energy we can see. They change the flow of energy in a space by intentional selection and assignment of furniture, or by specific placement of a decorative item. Another school, the Compass School, teaches the practitioner to go into a space with what is called a "Lao Pan" Compass (English spellings of all these Chinese terms vary). This compass is used to determine the directional influences on a property in relation to the universe in order to engage the Heaven Chi—the energy we cannot see.

Classical Feng Shui teaches that Heaven, Earth and Humanity energies need to be balanced to attain health and prosperity. These energies are called the "three gifts of energy" or the "San Cai." Since I am a visual person, I actually like to think of these feng shui energies as a sandwich. The top slice of bread is Heaven, the invisible Chi. The bottom slice is Earth Chi, the Chi we can see. In the middle is the human experience. The relationship between these three layers is the arena in which the feng shui practitioner orchestrates this artful science. The energies of heaven, humanity and earth must be manipulated so that all three interact with each other like a beautiful song. I believe that in order to balance the Chi energies of a property, the most thorough feng shui consultations use both Form School and Compass School strategies. To put it simply, without both the top and bottom slices of bread there is no sandwich!

The Five Elements

Throughout this book I will be referring to the word "element" or the term the "Five Elements." I would like to introduce you to these "Five Elements" so that you can fully grasp how they factor into my EcoChi concept.

Just as nature goes through cycles of change, so do we. We are the seasons, we are nature and we are the elements. In feng shui, the Five Elements are earth, metal, water, wood and fire. These elements are symbolic of the forces at work within the universe and how these forces impact our minds and bodies, as well as how they affect all other living creatures. The Five Element Theory is also the basis of Traditional Chinese Medicine, qigong practices for energy healing, and acupuncture-based therapy.

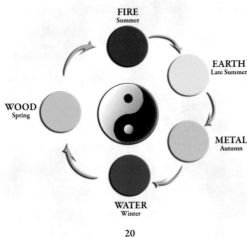

ENERGY CHARACTERISTICS OF THE FIVE ELEMENTS

	Color	Season	Direction	Weather	Personality
FIRE	Red	Summer	South	Heat	Passionate
EARTH	Yellow	Late Summer	Center	Thunder	Dependable
WOOD	Green	Spring	East	Wind	Expressive
METAL	White	Autumn	West	Cold	Precise
WATER	Black	Winter	North	Rain	Adaptable

Ancient Chinese philosophy teaches us that we have a measure of control over our lives and that by using feng shui techniques we can balance Chi and maximize good luck. However, it is generally agreed that feng shui only works if you are a person who also lives by this short list, which I have named "The Three Points of Honor." These are:

Educate yourself so that you have clarity in what you think and do;

Understand that we cannot control fate but can create opportunities; and

Undertake good deeds consciously, as an act of free will.

I advise my clients to check this short but profound list before, during and after incorporating EcoChi into their lives and projects. It is important that your core persona be aligned with these three principles, because they are vital to having the best human experience possible. If you do not live with honor, feng shui may not work at all, and certainly will not be as powerful and lasting.

21

The Green / Sustainability Factor

When you "Go Green and Sustainable" you have made choices that involve participating in an environmentally friendly lifestyle. The intention of these lifestyle choices and initiatives is to create ecological integrity by helping to protect the environment and sustain its resources for future generations. As I studied for my LEED® (Leadership in Energy and Environmental Design) exam, I soon realized how technically complex this subject is. LEED is a green building rating system and independent certification program that provides voluntary guidelines for developing energy-efficient, sustainable buildings. Created by the U.S. Green Building Council, LEED concentrates its efforts on improving performance across these five key areas:

- Energy efficiency
- Indoor environmental quality
- Materials and resources
- Sustainable site development
- Water quality and efficiency

In the course of my studies, I followed a rigorous regimen that included the close evaluation of all aspects of new and existing buildings, heating, ventilation and air conditioning systems, indoor air quality, landscape, neighborhood development, transportation, water quality and conservation, and more—including "brownfields." In the United States city planning jargon, a brownfield site is land previously used for industrial or commercial purposes. The land may be contaminated by low concentrations of hazardous waste or pollution, but still have the potential to be reused once it is cleaned up. Lands that require more substantial clean-up are not brownfields.

Misleading Use of the Term "Green"

During my months and eventually years of study in this new arena, I began to notice that many corporations, in their public communications, whether in the popular press or online, used the word green or even just the *color* green as a marketing tool. There is a term used to describe the deceptive use of green PR or green marketing. That term, "greenwashing," refers to the practice some companies employ of disingenuously spinning their products and policies to make them appear environmentally friendly when, in fact, they are not. As an informed consumer, your best way to make sure your dollars are buying and supporting safe, environmentally-conscious products, companies and practices is to carefully research all products you plan to use.

As my research and studies progressed, I also saw how integrating feng shui techniques could make Green spaces even better places to live in, work in or visit. With both of these disciplines in play, people within these environments would be more in harmony with the natural world, and live healthier and happier lives. This was all good, but for me something was still missing. I recognized that while I was being taught about energy efficiency, and how to reduce global warming, how to phase out ozone depleting chlorofluorocarbons, and new ways to save or make money by "going green," something big was still not being addressed, namely, the human experience!

Enter the Third Aspect of EcoChi:
Environmental Psychology

Environmental psychology is a fascinating, interdisciplinary science focused on fostering a greater understanding of the interplay between human beings and their environments. The field defines the term broadly; it can include natural environments, designed environments and learning, social and informational environments. It is believed that protecting, building and creating a "preferred environment" increases a sense of well-being in all human beings and facilitates behavioral effectiveness.

The questions addressed by this discipline are these: Do our homes, offices and public spaces make us feel peaceful, happy and sheltered? Do they feel like the safe havens they were meant to be? Are they calming, sustaining, mood-elevating and strengthening? All of this is attainable, and can be made possible with natural ventilation, lighting, plants, colors, shapes and views.

Looked at from a greater perspective, environmental psychology is about our relationship with Mother Earth. There are many different theories as to why we, as a species, have found ourselves seemingly intent on destroying our own planet. Some environmental psychologists believe that when we left our tribal way of living, we were separated from our mothers far too early in life. Under this theory, we experienced premature separation from the mother at the same time as we were being isolated from the natural world. This abrupt disconnection, the theory holds, has led us to suffer a kind of post-traumatic stress disorder. Underlying this hypothesis is the belief that feeling connected to the natural world is an essential component for proper maturing and responsible behavior toward the environment.

Others in this field hold that we as a species are suffering from a "disassociation syndrome." While similar to post-traumatic stress disorder and multiple personality disorder, this thinking is based on a belief that many, if not most, people are no longer able to respond appropriately to the natural world. The complex causes, as argued by the advocates of this particular theory, involve advertising, economic systems, politics, and our schools and universities, all of which reportedly have "disassociation" built into their fabric. Yet another theory is that humans may just be suffering from a form of collective amnesia. We have forgotten about our inherent link to nature and the lessons of our forefathers. If you want to look into this in depth, I encourage you to do your own research and draw your own conclusions. The more people who study this subject, the more aware we will all be. This can serve us as a society and bring us closer to living responsibly.

As I studied and undertook new projects, my findings took me by surprise. I could clearly see how environmental psychology could be integrated with feng shui and green and sustainable practices to enhance and deepen the human experience in our indoor spaces and in our world. Now I had my three-legged stool and EcoChi began to take shape.

As I said earlier, and it bears repeating throughout this book, what we look at, hear, taste, smell and touch influences our mood, our health, our success, our happiness and our future. Spaces that are birthed and bathed in the golden light of EcoChi create an inviting atmosphere and a place where people feel safe, secure and embraced.

A Ribbon of Light...

In the course of working with clients, it is sometimes beneficial to take them through a guided meditation. This is definitely not for everyone but it does have its place. Professional athletes often use this technique to visualize their goals, master their strategy, envision winning the championship, imagine what it would feel like and try to actually feel the sensation of the championship rings on their fingers. Much like an athlete, when you are busy running a business or dealing with a personal challenge, it can be difficult to empty your mind and clearly define your vision. The goals for your project or the next chapter of your life may be locked away inside of you. Utilizing meditation as one of my many tools is often the key that opens up clients to new ideas and a clear understanding of their own vision and goals.

To begin, I have them visualize a warm, healing, glowing golden energy that turns into a ribbon of light. With feet firmly on the ground, this glowing ribbon of light enters our bodies through the earth and travels through our organs. As it glows, it heals the intestines, liver, spleen, lungs and heart. This warm golden ribbon of light travels into our minds, and heals all of our emotions, stress and anxieties. The ribbon then travels through our heads and reaches to the heavens, thereby connecting us to all other energies and all possibilities as we become one with the universe.

This ribbon also runs through the EcoChi system. It is the link that interlocks the three major ingredients of this system—classical feng shui, green and sustainable living and environmental psychology—and puts us in the right frame of mind to nurture the environment, support our health and well-being and live up to our fullest potential.

It's been said before in many ways and has been attributed to Buddha, Confucius and others: "Wherever you go, there you are." EcoChi is built on the fundamental belief that "home" is wherever you are, and that it is essential to nurture your indoor space so that it nurtures the spirit within.

But how exactly does one do that? Let's move ahead to the front lines of people's lives, to see EcoChi in action and learn how it can provide you with the tools you need to enhance your life, both personally and professionally.

IF YOUR PARTNER'S SIDE OF

THE BED HAS A LARGER TABLE

THAN YOURS, IT OFTEN

MEANS THAT HE OR SHE IS

CARRYING MORE OF THE

RESPONSIBILITY IN THE

RELATIONSHIP.

✎ **Chapter Three**

Taking Life to a New Level

G rowing up in the sixties, I lived through the "Summer of Love" but never made it to Woodstock. Maybe I was a little too young or too afraid. So the culture of free love, drugs and rock and roll escaped me. At Queens College in New York, I studied communications and then, newly married at 19 years old, found myself working in my husband's family jewelry business.

The fine jewelry business was a visual wonderland! There were precious gems, along with glorious crystals that came in a wide range of colors, and all kinds of shiny precious metals. The colored stones fascinated me. I loved the infinite variety of their crystalline formations as well as the history, traditions and myths that surrounded them. At that time, most jewelers knew little about the stones they were selling. Eager to share my growing body of knowledge, I created a colored stone seminar for retail jewelers called "Romancing the Stone."

Many jewelers attended, excited to learn more about the gemstones that sat in their cases, glowing beautifully under the tiny spotlights. My seminars also attracted attention from department stores. Most of their salespeople had been transferred to fine jewelry from other departments, such as auto parts or home furnishings, so they were selling precious stone jewelry with no product knowledge or experience. One day their specialty was tires and the next day they were selling a bicolored watermelon tourmaline ring in 14 karat pink gold, with two .02 full cut diamonds on each side and a .08 total diamond weight. They were all hungry for information that would allow them to do a better job for their customers, and I was thrilled to supply as much detailed information as I could.

The successful reception of the seminars inspired me to learn even more, so I pursued a course of study at the prestigious Gemological Institute of America, earning my Graduate Gemologist degree. I am proud to say that I was also one of the first women to be certified by the American Gem Society.

My father-in-law, Clyde, served as my mentor. A genius at his work, he was a nurturing, loving and generous man as well as a highly creative designer. Working beside him, I learned not only about business, but also about life. He awakened my creative spirit by showing me how to turn a concept into a tangible reality. He intuitively knew that once you could envision something in your mind's eye, it was possible to actualize it. When something seemed difficult or even impossible I would ask him, "Dad, can we really do that?" His answer, *always,* was "Why not?"

In a way, that was my very first feng shui lesson, because feng shui teaches that what we picture in our imagination has the power to bring into our lives everything that we desire, and that the possibilities are endless.

That year, at the New York International Jewelry Show, I broke all of our company's sales records by taking the largest order we had ever written at that or any trade show. The next day, Clyde walked into my office with an ear-to-ear grin. I saw that he was carrying something large, flat and square, wrapped in brown paper. "I bought you something," he said. It was a print in a silver frame, depicting a foxhunt scene with a dozen or so men on horses, all in riding attire. In the forefront of the picture, already way ahead of her male competitors, rode a woman in a long dress and hat, her long hair flowing in the wind. The piece was entitled "My Lady Leads." "You left the guys in the dust," my father-in-law said. You were terrific!" He kissed me on the top of my head, then took out a hammer and picture hook and hung the picture on the wall directly in front of my desk. What I did not know at the time, but later learned, was that in feng shui this would be my "Red Bird." It was my father-in-law's confidence in me, exemplified by the picture he had placed on my wall that gave me the strength for my challenges and successes going forward. He knew that anything was possible if you could envision it, and he passed that confidence on to me—a wonderful gift I cherish and utilize in my work every day.

Enter Ann, a Fiery Redhead...

This is a Red Bird story. As I said earlier, all of the stories that follow are true. This one began with an e-mail I received from a woman named Ann, a "friend of a friend." A new member of a business organization to which I belonged, Ann wrote that she was very interested in feng shui, and also curious about my EcoChi system. She invited me to come to her apartment and begin working with her.

When I arrived at her home, I took a moment to quietly observe the space's energy. The first thing I felt was movement; there was a lot of activity in this apartment. There were beautiful paintings hanging on her walls, all of which depicted scenes of busy places filled with people having a good time. As I carefully studied her surroundings, I noticed that some furniture seemed out of place, like her oversized couch, which extended well into the small dining area. I also noticed stacks of books piled up on the floor and that a mound of clothing covered the seat and back of a living room chair.

Ann was a charming, pretty, energetic and highly intelligent woman. I could see the fire element in her eyes. She was dressed in black tights, a black tee shirt and pink running shoes. Her thick and wavy red hair was piled on top of her head with a clip, and when some loose strands occasionally fell on her face, she easily pushed the errant locks back into place. This was clearly a person who could take on the world and do it well! However, Ann was also somewhat guarded. Although she was very open with me about her plans to de-clutter and redecorate her apartment, the methodical way in which she described her plans, and the plans themselves, made it clear that her "emotional space" was well protected and under lock and key.

Ann lived in a one-bedroom condo. As we stood in the living room, she showed me a picture of the new couch she was about to order. I immediately recognized that that the couch would be way too big for the space. Ann also admitted that this apartment was supposed to be a temporary stop; she had never expected to live there for a long period of time. Although she had been there for three years, she admitted that the place somehow never felt like home.

I asked about her childhood and what home felt like back then. Her face lit up and her tone changed. Both her maternal and paternal grandmothers had played important roles in her childhood. They were warm, giving people. Both grandmothers served delicious meals in their homes. One loved to bake. Ann recalled the smell of fresh-baked bread in her Granny's kitchen. The family had sat around the table catching up on local gossip, laughing, sharing and enjoying a home-cooked meal. In Ann's past life, food = love = home. There was no way this apartment could feel like home when the living room furniture overlapped the dining area! There was not even a place for Ann to sit down to eat a take-out meal. If she could not manage to make room for a dining area, this apartment would never feel like her home.

After taking some compass readings and charting the feng shui energy, I found the "Ren Chi"—the heart of the home energy. It was located in the dining area and extended out to part of the living room. Now it would be my job to maximize this auspicious "Ren Chi" energy and help her to create the real home she deserved.

The first step was to choose a proper couch for the living room, one quite a bit smaller, with plush pillows for added comfort. With that kind of couch in place, she would have room for a dining table and chairs. And, since proper lighting is also very important for every room, I suggested dimmer switches, which would be a great tool for setting a distinct mood in each room while cutting down on energy use.

I also decided to place a mirror on the dining room wall. This, I explained to Ann, would double the heart energy and was part of how we were going to make the apartment feel like more than a temporary stop on her life's journey. The endgame was to allow Ann to finally feel like she had a home where she could enjoy herself, whether sitting down to a delicious meal by herself in a beautiful dining area, or dining with guests. I also suggested that she consider taking up baking as a new hobby—a suggestion she really liked.

When we got to the bedroom, Ann confided that she had been in a relationship for the past few years and was ready to take it to the next level and hopefully get married. However, this plan had hit a roadblock, since her boyfriend, Gary, was not receptive.

As I looked around the room, I told her that, in its natural and most powerful state, bedroom energy supports body regeneration and mental expansion. As you enter your bedroom, your energy, your Chi, should be transformed from your busy, daytime "yang" self to your restful "yin" self. The best sleep is when you feel as though you have left your body. This is the kind of sleep you often experience when you are on vacation in the mountains, by the sea or in the country. And ideally, that is how we are meant to sleep all the time.

Spoiling a Sacred Room

The bedroom is a sacred room. It is a private world for you and your spirit. There is also room for one other special person: your love partner. I asked Ann which side of the bed was hers and which was Gary's. I was somehow not surprised to see that right next to Gary's side of the bed was a desk with a computer, some of Ann's clothing and shoes, a pile of papers, and a large tri-fold mirror. Ann defended her use of that space for storage, explaining that because Gary had his own place, she felt free to use all the space for her personal items. After all, it *was* her apartment. Without comment, I looked under the bed and saw what was there. Together we pulled out her old cheerleading outfits from high school, love letters from a college boyfriend, a collection of stuffed animals, and a large plastic box that had one lonely noisemaker and paper hat from New Year's Eve 2000. Relics of an old life and an old love were still stuck under her bed. No wonder Gary was non-committal! It was high time to free it all up.

I talked to Ann about the energy beneath the bed and how she could unclog the channels of her romantic life by releasing the blocked energy that lay congealed under there. I also told her that storage under the bed can cause confusion, restlessness, allergies and sleepless nights. This room was seriously in need of attention. With EcoChi coming to the rescue, Ann's energy would be free to flow in a natural way, and as a result, she would become happier, healthier and closer to reaching her goals.

Another point I made to Ann that shocked her was the negative effect of her collection of stuff on Gary's side of the bed. It was made even more dramatic by the placement of the tri-fold mirror, which reflected Ann's possessions multiplied by three! What Gary saw when he came to visit, and what she herself looked at every day, were *her* things, magnified over and over again, making him feel less significant in her life, at least on a subconscious level. I am sure you have gotten the point, but let me emphasize: a bedroom with so many of one person's possessions in view leaves no room for a partner. I asked Ann to imagine that Gary had agreed to share his life in this apartment with her. Clearing out *his* side of the room would make room for *him* on an energetic level. To help her accomplish this, I suggested she purchase practical storage pieces that would hide her personal items from sight. I also asked her to move the desk away from his side of the bed. That desk, where it now was, represented her being "married" to her work, instead of being committed to—and making a priority of—the man in her life. If she truly wanted to change her life, she would have to change her priorities. Ann said she was more than willing to do so!

In big cities like Los Angeles, which is where she lives, light pollution is a stressor that can adversely affect our health and well-being because it interrupts the body's natural cycle. We need our rooms, and especially our bedrooms, to be dark at night. Nothing makes us healthier or sexier than a good night's sleep. For this reason I suggested blackout shades for this room.

We are all influenced by subliminal messages. The advertising business is alive and well because it works. When visiting Ann's bedroom I was aware of the messages she was sending to herself and those messages conflicted with her own goals and aspirations. I advised her to accent the bedroom in romantic colors, such as soft lavender and pink, because these colors have romantic Chi. Further, I suggested fresh cut flowers be placed in two identical vases. At the same time, I cautioned her that once the flowers began to wilt they must be thrown out immediately, because dying flowers or plants bring in a negative energy. Ann promised she would be vigilant about this.

In addition, I shared these techniques with her: If you are looking for a love partnership, or would like to enhance the romantic area of your life moving forward, decorate with pairs of things like the flower vases I suggested to Ann. Another example would be two candles in matching crystal candlestick holders. It is also important to have identical side tables on both sides of the bed, with identical lamps on each side as well. Couples need to even things out if they want a more balanced life. *What you see is what you get*, so if your partner's side of the bed has a larger table than yours, it often means that he or she is carrying more of the responsibility in the relationship.

Black Turtle Behind, Red Bird in Front

In the bedroom, the wall behind your bed is called your "Black Turtle." It is the "Mountain Chi," the energy that protects your back from unexpected danger—your support. As I mentioned earlier, the wall opposite the bed (or the wall you face from your desk or dining room table) is called the "Red Bird." In feng shui, this location is where your future is depicted. I always tell my clients to carefully choose what they put on this wall. It should represent what they want in their life—in other words, whatever their idea is of a bright future. That said, the very last thing I did in Ann's bedroom was to stand beside the headboard. I wanted to know what she looked at first thing every morning, and what the last thing was that she saw before she went to sleep. In essence, what did she now have as her "Red Bird?" This, by the way, was what Gary, her boyfriend and future-husband candidate, was also seeing, first and last, whenever he stayed over.

Ann's "Red Bird" was occupied by an original oil painting. As I looked at it closely, my mouth dropped open. It was a picture of a beautiful redheaded woman—in fact, one who looked a lot like Ann—sitting sadly alone staring at a telephone. Was she waiting for it to ring? I gently pointed this out to Ann, and suddenly she could no longer keep her emotions locked up. Her eyes welled up and a tear rolled down her cheek. I put my hands on her shoulders and kissed the top of her head. There was no need for words.

The next time I spoke with Ann she told me she had made all the changes I suggested, and was currently in the process of looking for a new piece of art, one that depicted lovers.

Three months later I followed up with Ann. She was very excited to hear from me. "Debra...oh Debra," she enthused, "I have so much to tell you! I found an incredible painting of lovers and was waiting for it to be delivered when Gary and I had a blowup. I decided our relationship was never going to lead to marriage so I told him it was over. Three days after the breakup, my painting arrived and I hung it on my Red Bird wall. The painting was nude lovers in an embrace. The next night I went out to meet some friends for dinner. I got there a little early, so I sat at the bar and ordered a glass of wine. This handsome man sat down beside me. We started to talk. We've have been seeing each other ever since. Guess what? He moved in this week and I have never been happier!"

I was blown away. But then her story got even better. "One day soon after that my friend Gail came to visit and meet my new boyfriend, David," Ann reported. She told me her friend came up to her apartment and asked to see the new painting in her bedroom. She loved the painting and asked where she and her husband could get one painted of the two of them. "After all, you and David look so happy in the picture," she explained.

The painting, of course, was not a portrait of Ann and David, although the likenesses were remarkable. Ann had not even met David until *after* she had bought the painting and it had been hung on her Red Bird wall. The universe—and EcoChi—certainly work in mysterious ways.

*PEOPLE WHO ACCUMULATE
LARGE AMOUNTS OF CLUTTER
MAY BE DEEPLY ATTACHED TO
ANOTHER TIME IN THEIR
LIVES—A TIME WHEN THEY
WERE HAPPIER, OR WHEN LIFE
SEEMED MORE MANAGEABLE.*

◆ **Chapter Four**

Sorting Through Chaos to Restore a Man's Castle

It was three o'clock on a Friday afternoon and I was sitting at my desk sipping a cup of green tea when I received a call from Steven. He phoned to ask if I could help his father. He sounded desperate and, in fact, admitted that he and his entire family were at their wits' end. Twelve years earlier, soon after Steven's mother died, his dad had suddenly become a hoarder. Henry began to buy all kinds of antique furniture and collectibles, and everything that came into the house stayed right there. This was especially alarming, Steven reported, because Henry was also constantly planning new construction projects around the house and purchasing supplies for them, even though none of them ever got started. Over the years, all these unused purchases had piled up everywhere. Steven also told me that, while he had repeatedly volunteered to help his father with his projects, the offers were always refused and nothing ever changed— except that the piles kept growing.

Sadly, the family felt they had no choice but to do something drastic—sell the property. First, though, they would have to seriously unclutter it. Steven wanted to know if I would be willing to drive out, look over the situation and see if I thought I could help. I told Steven I would be out the next day.

The drive to West Goshen, Connecticut took me on a beautiful route, and the area Henry lived in was filled with lovely homes on spacious acres of landscaped property. As I pulled into his driveway, I realized this was more than just a house; it was a mansion. Even though the grounds were run down, one needed little imagination to see that it had once been magnificent. And behind the house, sparkling in the sun, was a glorious silver and blue man-made lake that must have been about five miles long.

Henry greeted me at the front door. Towering at about 6'5", he was an elderly man with a lean build. I guessed him to be in his early eighties. That afternoon he was meticulously groomed in a clean shirt and jeans with a leather belt securing the pants around his slim hips. His full head of silver hair was wet, slicked back with water, and I could see a small black comb stuffed into the front pocket of his shirt. Despite his impressive appearance, something was brewing under the surface. As we shook hands, Henry's grip was firm. He was clearly trying to project confidence, but the slightly guarded way he looked at me through his metal-rimmed glasses projected trepidation, as if he was afraid I might be able to see right through him. All this happened in an instant, and I was more than ready to step over the threshold and see what the house had in store.

As Henry opened the front door to his mansion and stood back to let me in, I had to call on all my resources to show no outward reaction. I had seen clutter before, all levels of it, but the sight before me was almost unbelievable. There was everything you might expect to see in a severely cluttered home—the piles of newspapers, dirty dishes, cardboard boxes of all sizes, rusty tools, nails, screws, brackets, paintings, etc. But I was truly shocked to see two live chickens running across the great space, chicken-feed spread on newspapers on the floor and their droppings everywhere. Those chickens weren't the only surprise. I stopped counting at seven cats. One of them was blind, Henry calmly narrated, and one had only three legs. Overwhelmed by the chaotic sights, the smell of cat food, dirty litter boxes and chickens, I tried to hold my breath as I continued to follow Henry around the main floor.

It quickly became apparent that there was no place for a human being to sit—if one even wanted to sit down in that chaotic environment—because all of the furniture had piles of things covering every surface. As we entered the kitchen, I saw there was no room to cook a meal, since the room was littered with building materials on the counters, stove, in the sink and on the floor. I must have looked confused because Henry explained that his "next project" was a new kitchen for the basement! His thinking, he said, was that someday someone would buy this house and need a summer kitchen for outdoor entertaining. "After all, this house was made for entertaining," he added proudly. Entertaining aside, in truth, there was no room left in this house for Henry himself.

As Henry talked, I found him to be articulate, intelligent and charming. He also had a wealth of knowledge about the history of his property and this town that he had lived in for the past 25 years. As he spoke of other homes and public structures in and around the town, he rattled off the names of the architects, the years that the homes or buildings were built, their styles, the materials used, and more. Back on the home front, he had a compelling story to tell for each beautiful antique and piece of art he had collected over the years. He was a fascinating storyteller with a love and appreciation for his home and each piece in his various collections.

There was a major disconnect here, and the gap widened when Henry asked me what I thought he should attend to before putting his home up for sale, as his children were insisting he do. "Should I finish the downstairs kitchen or paint the living room?" he asked. "Or should I plaster the bedroom and update the bathrooms? Wait, maybe I should I put a new sculpture in the garden? Or search for a match to the antique molding in the library so it can be repaired? What do you think?" I thought of my own experience in packing up my home of twenty years as I was preparing to move after my divorce. At that time I had created the Stay-Maybe-Go System. That system had worked well for me, but instinct told me I would need a different tactic here. To help Henry solve his problem, I would have to successfully motivate him to free his home of all clutter. And in order to accomplish that, I would first have to earn his trust.

Holding On to a Happier Time

One tenet of modern psychology is that grief and guilt are common motivations for the uncontrollable acquisition and hoarding of objects. Those who accumulate the amount of clutter that Henry allowed in his home may be deeply attached to another time, place or person. People in these situations may have a strong desire to return to a better time—when they were happier, or when life seemed more manageable. Henry's hoarding began when he lost his wife. His abiding grief rendered him blind to what his house looked like, and how it was negatively impacting his life and the lives of his children.

When we sat down outside to talk and enjoy the fresh air, I began by addressing the new basement kitchen he had said he was planning to build. I could see that this project was a fantasy Henry had designed as a distraction. Brand new appliances, still in their boxes, were stacked in the kitchen, living room and dining room. I gently suggested returning these items and postponing the new basement kitchen until we finished renovating the main part of the house. To my surprise Henry readily agreed. He may have been secretly relieved, because he told me that he knew the kitchen project was a big job and he was, in fact, feeling a bit tired and not really up to it at the moment. So this was one thing he could cross off his to-do list!

Building on that not-so-small victory, I told Henry I was ready to answer his questions about where to start. We went back inside to discuss what needed to be done in the dining room, living room, library and den. Henry removed piles of papers from two dining room chairs and put the piles on the floor, allowing us to sit down to chat. I began by expressing my sincere appreciation for the property, its history, and the beautiful floors, moldings and original fireplaces. I also told Henry that there was no way I could tell him what project to start with until I could really *see* the rooms. How could I possibly help him choose a paint color for the walls if I could not see them? As far as what to do with the original floors, I said I could not see the condition of the wood because the floors were totally covered. So, where to start? I chose the room we were in, the dining room, because it had the least amount of clutter. As I left, with another warm handshake, this time with no trepidation behind his eyes, I said I would come back next month. If the dining room was indeed empty when I returned, as he promised it would be, we could choose paint colors, flooring and moldings. I knew that Henry's projects were his lifeline, so I could only hope he would rise to the challenge.

Happily, a month later I came back to find the room empty. Together we began refreshing and restoring the house—and indirectly his life—room by room. Henry fervently tackled the clutter in each room in anticipation of my next visit. He would say with a smile, "I hate you. Look at all the work you made for me." I would agree with him and smile right back.

As Henry's castle was slowly and methodically restored to its former splendor, his family's imperative to sell it was taken off the table. After all, this property was being transformed into a home where Henry could now live healthfully and happily.

A year and a half later, I received another phone call from Steven. It was holiday time and Henry wanted me to join his family, as their honored guest, to help them enjoy the first holiday dinner held in the mansion since his wife passed away. Steven said, "You gave my dad his life back. Thank you." I was just so glad I could help, but timing was a big factor in the success of this enterprise. Henry had been ready, and the teacher had appeared.

Understanding Clutter, and the Part it May Play in Your life

What is clutter anyway, and why do so many of us do this to ourselves?
CLUTTER, according to Princeton University's wordnet, is defined as:

1. A confused multitude of things

2. Filling a space in a disorderly way

3. Unwanted echoes that interfere with the observation of signals on a radar screen

I especially love that last definition, "unwanted echoes that interfere with the observation of signals on a radar screen." That is an insightful metaphor.

Clutter is an ailment that affects our society as a whole, and is both a direct and an indirect result of our rampant consumerism. Rather than continue the adolescent behavior that echoes the chant of "The one who dies with the most toys wins," it is time for more of us to make mature, responsible choices that benefit both ourselves and our world. Let's create the next chic trend by transitioning from "More, More and More" to "Less Is More!"

With EcoChi, I show people how, when they are surrounded by clutter, they often miss the following important *signals,* which, like an undiagnosed illness, are actually symptoms of more significant issues that need to be dealt with. Are you missing the "dangerous clutter" signals in your life?

Signal #1
You buy things that you don't really need and then have to find places to put them.

Clutter is a common ailment in our consumerist society. Advertisers tap into the emptiness we feel inside by tempting us with new products that overtly or subtly promise to make us feel better. We buy what they are selling and then realize that the thing we bought does not and cannot make us happy. This sets us up for our next purchase. But the next new item holds only more empty promises, and the vicious cycle continues.

Signal #2
You have reached a point in your business or personal life where you feel stuck.

Clutter produces confusion for those who live or work in a disordered, jam-packed space, and leaves no room for new and wonderful things to come into their lives. Organize your life and you automatically ramp up the functionality of your home and office. By throwing away the *echoes* of your past you make room for the *signals* that, once you heed them, will lead you to the infinitely brighter future that awaits you: a future that might be just one dumpster away!

Signal #3
You have developed allergies and other health issues.

Are you suffering with breathing problems, a stuffy nose or watery eyes? Clutter is a breeding ground for vermin, pests, mold and mites, which can create all kinds of health risks and allergies. It can also lead to unpleasant odors that even when masked with scented sprays or candles can adversely affect the enjoyment of one's space. Reorganizing your space will bring in a breath of fresh air in more ways than one.

Signal #4
The areas of your office or home overflow from one room into another.

This kind of loss of boundaries indicates that the space is under anxious tension. For example, if papers and other items from your home office have overflowed onto your dining room table and your living room couch, this clearly reflects an unbalanced life. In feng shui, items piling up in a disorganized fashion are believed to be a heart attack in the making. De-cluttering opens up the passages and allows healthy Chi to flow through your rooms and your life.

Signal #5
You avoid inviting people into your home or office.

Clutter keeps people out! In a cluttered space there is simply no room for socializing or effective business interactions. You may even be ashamed of your messy place and not invite anyone in. This can dramatically limit your ability to establish fulfilling, enriching and socially or financially profitable relationships. When everything is neat, clean and in its rightful place, you are infinitely more likely to invite and receive more great people, success and prosperity into your life.

Signal #6
You are holding onto a happier time by keeping things far beyond their expiration date.

Remember 15 years ago when you were three sizes smaller? It is human to keep hoping to fit into those clothes someday, but not practical or smart. Think of what you will gain by donating them to appreciative people who can use these garments today. A clutter-free environment, including less cramped closets and drawers, will give you room to create unexpected and rewarding new opportunities.

Signal #7
You have a busy life in which there is no time to put things away, so you leave piles to go through "later"—a later that never comes.

Whether it's piles of mail, clothing or anything else you leave lying around, at the end of the day it takes much more time to go through piles of things than it does to put them in their proper place immediately. Later, tomorrow, next week, "soon" almost never comes, because life keeps throwing more challenges at you that you need to keep up with on a daily basis. Staying organized is a deliberate habit you need to cultivate till it becomes second nature. Do that, and I promise you will discover that this will make you feel much more in control of your life.

Clutter can "put the brakes on" when it comes to your personal goals and your career. It can clog up the veins of your life and prevent money, love, health and happiness from flowing in. It's not just about the past; it's is about making room for your future.

I am here to tell you, from my own experience, that de-cluttering is not easy. But nothing worthwhile is ever easy. I did it, and so can you! At the end of the next chapter, I will share with you some of my favorite tips for removing clutter that can help you make it through the process with a minimum of angst.

UNDERSTANDING WHAT

CAUSES PEOPLE TO BECOME

RESTLESS IN SPACES, I ALREADY

HAD AN IMPORTANT CLUE

AS TO WHAT JESSICA'S

PROBLEM COULD BE...

Chapter Five

An Office in the Sky Gets a Major Overhaul

O ver time, I have come to understand that each of us is motivated and driven by a fundamental underlying force. My personal motivation was a difficult childhood. Fortunately, I was able to find a safe, nurturing haven in school, and also at the public library. Books were my first love and, in those early years, the library became my second home. The stories I read were a great escape, and they created wonderful possibilities for a better life ahead, in my mind and in my soul. At home I wrote poems and essays in my personal journal. At age nine, I wrote my first poem, which I called "A Room with Four Walls." I still ache for the little girl inside me who wrote these words: "I am enclosed in a room with four walls, with nobody in it but me. Someone take me from this place. I am helpless... set me free."

Even at that young age, I had a strong need for a room to be more than four walls. I wanted then what I want even more now—for the spaces each of us inhabit to be healthy environments that nurture the human spirit, that keep us in rhythm with Mother Nature, and that act as catalysts to bring about the life we want and deserve. Still, I had periods in my personal and business lives when I was stuck. Some of these experiences could have destroyed my life. Instead, they were the impetus to find solutions and redefine my path. None of it was easy—which is why Jessica's plight so resonated with me.

Jessica's All Too Common Dilemma

Jessica heard me speak at a business conference in upstate New York and was curious as to what EcoChi could do for her business. She asked me to visit her office in Manhattan on a Sunday when no one was around so that she could give me her complete attention. The recession was taking its toll on her company, and she was struggling to keep it afloat. She also complained about a feeling of restlessness when she was in her office. She found it difficult to focus there. Jessica actually preferred to take her work down to a local café. She was able to work there for hours and get so much more accomplished than at her desk. Understanding what causes people to become restless in spaces, I already had an important clue as to what Jessica's problem could be, and was eager to see if my instincts were correct.

At age 34, Jessica was the founder and CEO of a successful marketing company that she had started eight years before. After her third year in business, she had brought in a partner named Stacy to help manage the company's growth. Stacy was charged with handling the internal day-to-day running of the business, while Jessica was the outside person, selling their marketing services and developing new clients.

In 2007, when the recession began, businesses immediately reduced their budgets, and marketing was the first expenditure to go. Jessica found she had to cut back on her own company expenses, rethink her business plan, and find creative ways to adapt her business to the unpredictable economic environment.

I met her in the lobby of her office building and rode the elevator to her offices, which were on the 35th floor of a luxury building with stunning panoramic city and Central Park views. Jessica is a blonde, blue-eyed beauty. Even when dressed conservatively in a pants suit and man-tailored blue shirt, she could not hide her shapely figure. It was clear throughout our conversation that she was charming, intelligent and perceptive. Now I had to figure out why she was feeling so unfocused in her office, and why she was struggling to maintain the success for which she had worked so long and so hard.

On her floor we walked past the reception area and then past another three rows that each contained three desks. There was also a common conference room and four private offices, all of which ran along large picture windows. As Jessica led me into her private office, a helicopter flew right by the window. She actually waved to the pilot. Impressive as this was, I soon realized that this dramatic sight was nothing compared to the ride I was about to take *her* on.

Jessica's desk faced a wall, and on either side of the desk stood metal storage cabinets six feet high by five feet wide. The desk itself was covered with layers of newspapers, clipped articles, folders, open and unopened mail and three packages of chewing gum. I also counted five photo frames, all of different sizes, shapes and colors. The pictures, she told me, were of nieces, nephews and herself with an old boyfriend skiing in Aspen. There was also a framed photo of her beloved cat, Tammy.

Jessica asked me to sit down, but the seat of the one side chair was covered with goodie bags from past conferences and charity events. On top of the bags were several granola bars and a couple of CDs. Jessica quickly grabbed the whole pile and laid it on top of the fax machine. Why she got more work done out of the office was no longer a mystery.

As we talked, I asked her some questions about her goals, and Jessica told me about her new business plan. She said she was excited to break into social networking—a new area for her business. One immediate challenge was that this was something her partner did not want to explore. In fact, Stacy saw no reason to make any changes to their business. However, the advice from her accountant, and her own assessment of the situation, convinced Jessica that if she did not make some adjustments quickly, they would go out of business. That thought terrified her, she admitted, since she had gone down that painful road once before. Her first business, a gourmet popcorn wholesale company, had failed within 18 months.

I looked around carefully. It was clear to me that *any* change would be for the better. First, Jessica's desk was facing a wall, while her back was to the door, which is a big feng shui no-no. That I would deal with later on. Nothing could be moved or changed until we took care of the biggest problem of all, the clutter. I asked Jessica what was in her storage cabinets. She told me that they were filled with important documents. One had papers, records, files and old checkbooks from the popcorn business. The other file cabinet held old tax returns, old business plans and strategies, and files from closed accounts—meaning clients who no longer used her marketing services.

Towers of Terror Hold Jessica Back

What was clear to me, though not yet to her, was that, even more important than the "stuff" that was in her cabinets was what the stuff *represented*. The detritus in her metal file cabinets was a large part of what was holding Jessica back. Those huge, towering storage areas on either end of her desk were weighing her down, closing her in and keeping her from reaching her goals. During this difficult economic time, Jessica needed to unburden herself and her business of the past, and move forward by making room for new and exciting changes.

On the home front, a bedroom filled with clutter often causes insomnia.

In an office, clutter causes restlessness and an inability to focus on the tasks at hand. Restlessness at work is, in fact, universally symptomatic of a clutter problem. Clutter creates very fast moving and erratic Chi, which in turn causes an uneasy feeling. This is what makes it difficult to concentrate. My first suggestion was to move the storage cabinets into the spare office. Once these "Towers of Terror," as I called them, were gone, it would be easy to turn the desk around so that Jessica could stop looking at a blank wall, which symbolizes a dead end. Instead, once we turned her desk around, Jessica would be sitting in a power position. With a wall behind her, which is the mountain energy, she would have the necessary support for her endeavors moving forward. In this position she would also be able to see the door of her office, which would bring her a greater sense of control and power. When she could look out of the window, literally and figuratively, she would face an endless horizon of future possibilities for her business (her Red Bird).

Jessica was open to these suggestions, and told me she would get the building's handyman in to help her move those file cabinets the very next morning. For now, we would go down to the nearby office supply store and buy appropriate desk organizers. This we did, and returned to set up the Stay-Maybe-Go System for the items on, in and around her desk, and even for the massive pile now sitting on top of the fax machine. All articles, folders, random papers and magazines designated for the Maybe pile were put into a carton. I had Jessica date the Maybe box with a permanent marker. We then moved that box into the spare office.

I told Jessica I was going to call her in three months to see how things were going, and that at that time any papers from that Maybe box that had not been read, referred to or otherwise used would be moved to the Go pile to be shredded and recycled. I also asked her to toss out the picture of her with her old boyfriend. We also replaced all the mismatched frames with just three matching photo frames, and put pictures in them that represented how she wanted her life to look in her soon-to-be bright future. Of course her beloved feline Tammy made the cut!

On Monday, Jessica called to ask, in what was clearly a last ditch attempt to retain the status quo, if it would be okay to turn her desk around, but still leave the two big file cabinets in place. I told her that as long as she held on to the past there would be no room for her new business ideas to take off. "No, Jessica," I said, "You cannot leave the Towers of Terror in your office. Sorry, but they have to go!"

Three weeks later Jessica left me a voice message. "I moved both cabinets into the spare office and turned my desk around, and it feels great!" She is now productively working at her uncluttered desk and only goes to the local café for an occasional breakfast meeting. She has brought in several new clients, is actively building her social networking business and has even reclaimed several established customers with her new service. Jessica realized that there were such insurmountable differences in their visions for their business, and began the process of buying Stacy out of the partnership. Overall, this remarkable business owner's office is now the entranceway to a bright new future.

Steps to Unclutter Your Spaces

For those who are very organized by nature, it may seem like this chapter is a big deal about nothing. However, you would be surprised at how many people struggle with the clutter in their lives. I have created simple steps for those who are too close to the problem to see the solution.

When tackling clutter, it is easy to get discouraged and overwhelmed before you even start. Here are ten practical tips I offer my clients, which have proven useful to them. I suggest you start by trying out one—whichever is easiest for you. When you finish, congratulate yourself! Then set a date for the following week to tackle another. Before you know it, you will have cleared out all the clutter that is past its expiration date and subconsciously holding you back. As greater abundance enters your life, you will discover how powerful this fresh new energy is.

Ten Tips for an Uncluttered Home or Office Space

1. Every time you buy something new, throw or give away one item you do not use. This will keep you on an even playing field. Even better, toss or donate *two* things every time you bring in something new. This will keep you on the right road. Remember: Cultivate an attitude that Less is More!

2. Get serious. Take a day for just this. Begin by making three piles. Stay-Maybe-Go! Put the Maybe pile in a carton. Date the carton and then put it in some form of storage for six months. Before you open it up again, make a list of all the things in the box that you may have wanted and truly missed. Keep only the things on that list. The rest has to GO!

3. Buy containers to organize everything you want to keep and create neat, tidy places for everything you own.

4. Store similar things together. For your office: put all paperclips in one clip holder, put Post-its in their proper place, put all files in the file cabinet, separated into two categories: current and closed business or clients. If you are doing this for your home, pair all socks in the sock drawer and throw out the singles. Organize all tools in the toolbox, recipes in your recipe box, and make sure your utensil drawer is neat.

5. When you take your clothes off at the end of the day, hang them up and throw anything to be laundered into the laundry basket. It takes time to sort through clothes or press clothing that would likely have not gotten wrinkled if you hung it in the closet in the first place. Doing this right away will save you precious time later on.

6. Throw junk mail away as it comes in, remembering to recycle paper items. Bills go in the proper tray or basket, and interesting reading material goes in the Maybe pile. If you do not read it within a month, you are never going to read it, so then, out it goes.

7. Make your first project a small one to avoid overwhelming yourself. There is no need to become anxious. You can de-clutter one drawer, one closet, one side of the room at a time. If you keep at it regularly, you will soon have a handle on the entire situation.

8. Take a photo or video of items you don't really need but for whatever reason feel uneasy about giving or throwing away. This is a way to have it forever without allowing it to take up valuable room and "clog the arteries" of your life.

9. Make a list of all the positive things that will be created for your life in a clutter-free environment. This can include better health, a deeper, more refreshing night's sleep, improved mood, better relationships, more space, more time, no late fees on your bills, easier management of office and home, and much more room for new things and people to enter your life.

10. When the job feels too big to handle on your own, think about hiring a professional organizer. Sometimes paying for a service is all the motivation a person needs. Most professional organizers get paid by the hour. Of course, once the professional finishes setting the system up you must make a commitment to keep all systems organized, or you will soon find yourself back in the same chaotic situation.

Change is never easy, and I applaud you for your willingness to get started and to keep at it. I will also say that the challenge is even greater and the stakes higher when we deal with those things we cannot see but can still harm us. Many of our indoor spaces are filled with toxins that affect our health and well-being. Unfortunately, much of the time we are clueless about the fact that these dangers even exist, and thus have no idea of their negative effects. In the next chapter we'll take a look at how we can ensure that our homes and offices—or any spaces we occupy—are safe and healthy places for us to be.

Each of us has the power within our own bodies, minds and environments to heal ourselves from a variety of ailments. The turning point from illness to wellness could be something we source from inside or the outside.

In Healthy Design, Be Especially Wary of "Poison Arrows"

We are energy, and so are all of the things around us, both animate and inanimate. Invisible but powerful patterns of energy exist everywhere. This is the basic principle of quantum mechanics, which has been observed and documented by scientists at the scale of atomic particles. All matter has this "Chi" energy or "life force." What's important to note for the purposes of this chapter is that some energy patterns are supportive, even restorative to health. Others can be destructive, and can make us ill in body, mind or both. Energy patterns are affected by a great many factors, all working in tandem. This can include the colors and shapes we choose, the positioning of furniture, the lighting, the floor plan, the site, and even the size and location of the doors and windows. The way the space will be utilized also factors in as does its history, whether it's a home, office, hotel room, movie theatre, or any other location. What has happened in that space? Was someone sick? Did someone die there? Were toxic paints, materials, finishes or adhesives used in building or renovating the property? Was there love in that space, or violence and anger? So many variables enter into the equation, including the basic fact that energy is always in a state of flux. Once you become sick, for example, your home, office or other space may have unstable energy that can hinder your recovery, or even lead you to a relapse. For this reason, making sure a space has good nurturing energy, enhancing that positive energy, and, when necessary, containing or eliminating the stressful energy, is an essential part of the EcoChi process.

Ronnie and the "Poison Arrows"

Each of us has the power within our own bodies, minds and environments to heal ourselves from a variety of ailments. The turning point from illness to wellness could be something we source from inside or the outside. Sometimes it's a prescription, a diet change, a homeopathic remedy, care by a traditional western trained doctor, an acupuncturist, a sound healing session, prayer, meditation or EcoChi-inspired adjustments made to a space. These are all valid treatments or preventative alternatives. The following client experience is a perfect example of how our surroundings impact our health.

The setting was Marina Del Ray, California, where I visited a sprawling new residential apartment. I had been asked to bring EcoChi to a well-known television journalist I will call Ronnie. As she opened the door to welcome me into her home, I looked over her shoulder and saw the Pacific Ocean glistening through her living room windows, which ran floor to ceiling and from one end of the apartment to the other. A gorgeous 30-something woman with long dark hair and piercing black eyes, Ronnie was dressed in straight-legged, skintight jeans that accentuated her long legs and athletic build, a white tunic top, small gold hoop earrings and black ballerina flats. She had a sincerity and earthiness about her, yet projected such rare elegance that I felt as though I was in the presence of royalty.

As she puttered around her immaculate kitchen, making me a delicious cappuccino, Ronnie talked about her work. She related how at any time, even in the middle of the night, she could get a call and, at a moment's notice, have to pack a bag and fly out to the Middle East or some other far-off destination where news was being made. She had been doing this for over a decade and had come to accept this as a way of life. With eyes looking down and fidgeting with an earring, Ronnie took a moment to tell me that she was deeply grateful for how well compensated she was for her work and how, because of that, money was never a concern. I picked up a hint of guilt in her mannerisms; she almost seemed to be apologizing for her success.

After our cappuccino and chat, I asked her to give me a tour of the space. The architectural style of the 3 bedroom, 3 ½ bath apartment was straightforward.

With windows galore, it was primarily designed to feature the breathtaking ocean views and sunsets. But all was not perfect in this seemingly idyllic setting. Returning to the living room, I noticed two "poison arrows," which took the form of two faux walls meeting at very sharp angles. Her floor plan indicated where her new couches were going to be placed and I was not happy with the proposed layout. The sharp edges of the walls were going to be pointing right at Ronnie when she entertained or when she was home alone, just relaxing on one of the couches. I explained to Ronnie that that these were "poison arrows" and that the sharp angles would cause fast moving "Sha Chi," which would make her and her guests feel restless and uncomfortable in the living room. This inauspicious energy could also negatively impact her health and well-being. Try to be aware of this in your own life. The next time you feel uncomfortable in a space look around you; maybe it is a poison arrow that is causing the problem.

This information was troubling to Ronnie, and she looked quite upset when I expressed my concerns. As it turns out, this *was* the one room that she did not feel comfortable in. She then lowered her voice almost to a whisper, and confided in me that she had experienced some unexpected health challenges over the last couple of years. She was certain these issues were environmentally-induced. After all, she was young, health-conscious, and kept herself in fit condition. My heart went out to her because I can understand how disappointing it is when your body betrays you. I told her that these sharp "poison arrows" simply had to be eliminated from the architectural plan!

We set up another appointment where I met with her architect, Gene. At first he said that he did not want to put up curved walls as I suggested; he felt it would compromise the integrity of the architectural design. Fortunately, Ronnie insisted that the walls be curved. So Gene and I created a design with curved walls. We included a large cutout in both of the walls. Each would house a sculpture, complete with built-in lighting for accent and mood. This would eliminate any sharp corners from the living room area, slow down the Chi, and create a "Sheng Chi" (good energy) in that living room. Now Ronnie would be surrounded by beauty inside and outside, with no poison arrows compromising her health and well-being. She was delighted!

Having learned about Ronnie's medical history, it was imperative for me to address all her health concerns regarding the planned renovation she was about to undertake. This is where my training as a professional LEED Green Associate is an essential tool for designing spaces. Ronnie needed more than design advice, more than energy mapping, and more than ways to attract good fortune. With her bright, inquisitive mind, she also needed help to understand the science behind the construction and remodeling she was about to live through. What kind of stress (Sha Chi) was she about to create in her new space during and after she renovated, painted and refurnished?

Ronnie, like most people I work with, had never heard of volatile organic compounds (VOCs). VOCs are the gasses that are emitted and released into the air by a wide range of products, including paints, lacquers, adhesives, carpets and even furniture. These substances all emit VOC compounds. In fact, due to high levels of VOCs, indoor pollution can be up to five times worse than outdoor pollution. I was particularly concerned about Ronnie's bedroom. It is there that she, like most of us, spends 6 to 8 hours a night sleeping, which is the restorative time our bodies use and need to stay healthy. What airborne toxins would she be inhaling even while she slept? Unlike "poison arrows," volatile organic compounds are invisible, but they can be lethal.

I soon realized that I was overwhelming Ronnie with information so I made a checklist of all the things I wanted her to think about before she gave her renovation the green light. Ronnie now had the ammunition necessary to ask the right questions and take charge of her life. I have included this list for any readers who are contemplating their own building or renovation projects. If you know what your options are, you can make healthier, more informed choices. Please be your own health advocate and, in so doing, create "Sheng Chi" for *your* space!

Checklist for a Healthy Bedroom

✓ Do you always choose low or no VOC paints? There are many healthy paint choices today, so do your research. There are even beautiful milk paints to consider, in yummy colors!

✓ What kind of carpeting are you choosing for the bedroom? Natural materials like wool, silk, cotton, hemp or bamboo fiber are becoming readily available.

Choose organic whenever possible, and ask if the material was chemically treated in any way. If it was, move on!

✓ Are the adhesives being used to install the carpeting "Green Label Plus" approved? This means they were tested by a third party and are a healthier choice for you and for the planet.

✓ What kind of headboard is a good choice for your bed? A solid wood headboard is the best "Black Turtle" (protective energy). It also acts as a barrier between you and any electrical wires or plumbing in the walls. Be sure that the wood you use is certified by the Forest Stewardship Council or an equivalent independent, nonprofit organization that promotes responsible management of the world's forests. Also check to be sure that any finish on the wood has low VOCs and is formaldehyde-free.

✓ Have you considered how your bedding impacts your health? If you want a peaceful night's sleep, eight hours spent in an organic, pesticide-free environment certainly is a choice worth considering. For extra health benefits and comfort, shop for an all-natural latex mattress. Stay away from metal coils, because they conduct electromagnetic fields, and also conduct the radio frequency waves that are emitted from electric equipment and appliances.

✓ Are the electronics in the bedroom plugged into a surge protector? This is an easy way to save money on energy bills by preventing "energy vampires," which are the electronic appliances that use energy even when turned off. A surge protector will reduce your exposure to radio frequency waves and electromagnetic fields. Studies show these emissions interrupt sleep and can cause health problems. For a restful night's sleep and a lower energy bill, simply shut off the main switch on the surge protector before you go to bed.

✓ Do you have any "poison arrows" in your space? These sharp angles cause energy to move faster and can make you restless, interrupt your sleep, and negatively impact your health. Soften these edges with plants, wind chimes or decorative screens. This added beauty brings a positive quality to your experience of the space while slowing down the Chi—all of which makes for a healthier environment.

I visited Ronnie soon after she moved into her newly renovated apartment. She was delighted with the end result; she was sleeping well and felt remarkably healthy again in her new home. "Every time I see my curved walls and beautiful sculptures, I think of you and the wonderful changes you have brought into my life," she said. Then Ronnie gave me what I consider the highest compliment. She used the Sanskrit greeting that translates "I honor the Spirit in you which is also in me": "Namaste, Debra." With a nod of my head and hands held together in a fashion of prayer, I returned the greeting with a smile and a full heart.

In Healthy Design, Be Especially Wary of "Poison Arrows"

The world is getting "greener." As we implement LEED®, green practices and sustainability in all aspects of our lives, these practices are steadily becoming the new standard.

✆ Chapter Seven

Hotels and Public Spaces: Think in Curves

The Chief Architect of our world clearly loves curves. Picture the swirls and curls of the ocean waves, the gentle arc of a flower petal, the perfection of a full moon, or the spiral motion of caressing winds on a balmy evening. There is a lesson here, one I learn over and over again as I work in grand spaces such as hotels, retail stores, convention centers, restaurants or office buildings.

I learned it anew while working on the redesign of a hotel lobby. My assignment was to recreate the atmosphere in the lobby so guests would want to spend more time there and use it as a meeting place, instead of what they had been doing—gathering outside the hotel. It was important to the owner that people linger in the lobby because it was connected to the bar area, restaurant and gift shops, all of which had great potential as profit centers for his hotel.

As I walked through the lobby, I noted the tall vertical columns that were on either side of a common seating area, anchoring the space. The area was attractive, but was also formal and somewhat forbidding. The owner wanted this seating area to be more than a showplace. He wanted it to also serve as a friendly space with a feeling of community, an area where hotel guests actually congregated. What I saw, however, was an entire lobby designed with boxy, intersecting lines. Everything, including the chairs, side tables and lighting fixtures, was designed either in squares, rectangles or triangles. These polygons were everywhere, and were far from inviting.

Having only straight lines and sharp angular shapes in our personal and public spaces is like being in a room full of arrows of different sizes and colors that point straight at us, from all directions and heights. Not surprisingly, this kind of environment will make us feel uncomfortable, nervous and agitated.

Some people are more sensitive than others to their surroundings and, in particular, to "poison arrows." Those who are extremely sensitive will feel as though they cannot wait to leave the space. Some people, when experiencing "Sha Chi"—negative energy—even get chills or goose bumps and display anxious behavior. A common symptom would be someone nervously glancing at his or her watch repeatedly. You may hear something like, "I really can't stay, I have an early meeting in the morning." In truth, they really can't stay! These people are reacting to their environment with an instinctive, unconscious urgency. They know they have to get out but, with their reaction coming from a subconscious level, they don't exactly know why.

Those who are less sensitive may just feel somewhat restless, unable to focus, or vaguely uneasy. This was the experience of many of the hotel's guests. Most of them clearly preferred standing in front of the entrance, gazing at the beautiful park across the street, rather than doing what the hotel owner and management would have preferred—staying inside, relaxing and spending money in an inviting environment.

The perfect EcoChi solution for this hotel owner's problem was to slow down the Chi in the lobby, which is exactly what we did. I incorporated gentle bows and circles in this space, and replaced some of the furniture with pieces that embraced curves. For example, I created sitting areas with round tables and U-shaped chairs—chairs shaped like a hug.

I also found an amazing local architect who put together a team of craftsmen. They enthusiastically transformed the rectangular columns into cylinders that resembled tree trunks. Then, picking up on the park theme from across the street, I filled the lobby with native plants, adding life force energy to the space. The plants I chose naturally purified the air, absorbed electromagnetic fields emanating from electronics, slowed down Chi, and added color and the "wood element," which symbolizes freshness and new beginnings. These were all giant steps forward in keeping hotel guests happy and secure while offering them a subtle but very real sense of well-being.

We also added arched entrances to the room, as well as round planters and lighting fixtures designed with gentle curves. Sheng Chi" (good energy) was now moving throughout, creating a harmonious and nurturing atmosphere where people wanted to linger.

Of course, there were other factors to consider. I continued to enhance the human experience in this hotel by addressing lighting, ventilation, temperature, fragrance, sounds and views. I also addressed the offgassing of building materials and furnishings—in other words, I kept VOCs under control so the releasing of chemicals into the air adversely affecting the indoor air quality was limited.

The end result of the EcoChi redesign of this lobby was that the community embraced the hotel as an extension of the park across the street. It is now a popular meeting place for hotel guests and city residents alike. Revenues have increased in the retail areas, bar and restaurant due to increased traffic, as people now choose to spend leisure time in the lobby—much to the delight of the hotel owner.

Spaces That Make Us Feel Connected, Comfortable, Alive...

Connecting with the natural world gives us a more peaceful feeling. Close to the heartbeat of the universe, you can't help but feel part of something bigger, whether it is the tides, the seasons or the cycles of life. Bringing the outdoors inside makes people happy. Happy guests spend more money, make frequent visits and recommend your facilities to others. Likewise, employees who are happy take fewer sick days, work longer hours and smile more often. This is how to make your guests even happier and, at the same time, increase your ROI.

What makes us want to return to certain places? Even when we cannot go back, there are places that have taken hold and live within us. We will happily and enthusiastically share our memories of them with friends, family and colleagues. Those are the types of memories you want your spaces to evoke. There are places that I personally hold dear in my memory bank, will never forget and will always long to return to. These cherished locations include Bar Harbor Maine's Acadia National Park with its sorbet-colored sunrise, where from the top of the mountain you can see both the Atlantic Ocean and a freshwater lake. Another is the Sculpture Garden at the Museum of Modern Art in Manhattan—specifically on an autumn day, as the smell of roasted chestnuts from the street vendors fills the air.

For you it could be that special little restaurant on a side street in Rome. Maybe you sat at an outdoor table sipping cappuccino, serenaded by the soft background sounds of a fountain in the distance, as you spent the day watching people pass by. Perhaps it was the open air theater in Santa Fe, where the operatic music seemed to wake up every star in the night sky and lifted your soul. Maybe it was your favorite café in Venice Beach, CA—your own little secret place, where you ate a delicious vegan meal and awakened your creativity by writing, drawing or just daydreaming for hours. Take a minute to think of some of your own special places and make a list of the attributes that make those spaces so appealing to you. Implement some of the listed features into your own environment and allow the transformation to begin!

Another of my most favorite places is a spa in upstate New York. It is on Native American land and has an almost tangible spiritual energy. I found it by accident. I had signed up for a women's business conference run by the Women's Leadership Exchange, a major national connections-building organization. The weekend promised to be fascinating, since I would be spending quality time with other women business owners, sharing ideas and business solutions. What I noticed was how happy the attendees were. They loved spending time in the hotel lobby, where they had discovered several snug, warm, informal areas in which to network, chat or just relax. Everyone commented on how they loved the space. With my professional eye, I could see exactly why they all experienced the space in this way. The design embraced both Heaven (symbolized by circles) and Earth (symbolized by squares) in the most harmonic way. Everyone who walked into this lobby just wanted to sit down and spend time there.

What specific elements made this upstate spa so appealing? This is my list of the "Sheng Chi" (good energy) characteristics that were implemented in this particular property:

Some Characteristics of Sheng Chi

1. Glass walls with views of the garden and an outdoor fountain

2. Indoor plants and trees

3. Fireplaces with small seating areas that create cozy little nooks

4. Large skylights with views of the clouds, moon, stars and sun

5. Furniture positioning that made for a wonderful Chi flow

6. Colors that created a feeling of calm, especially beiges, greens and turquoise

7. Chairs and couches made of all natural materials. They were deep, over sized and more than comfortable; they were cozy. Most were U-shaped so it was like sitting in a warm, embracing hug.

8. The interplay between squares and circles was at a perfect balance, each flirting with each other in different places throughout the lobby and hall ways. The carpet was designed with a large square in front of every door way. This slowed down the Chi, and in so doing, created a proper Ming Tang (entranceway) for every guest.

9. The Five Elements were in balance through these components:

Fire: Fireplaces and the use of the color orange
Earth: Stone fireplace fronts, large rocks used in the garden, squares in art pieces
Metal: Metal Sculptures displayed in lobby area and garden
Water: Fountains visible from the seating area, a waterfall in the entrance, the use of turquoise in the art and in the lobby's jewelry display cases
Wood: Large, tall green indoor plants and views of the green garden and trees

Sustainability and Indoor Public Spaces

The world is getting "greener." As we implement LEED, green practices and sustainability in all aspects of our lives, these practices are steadily becoming the new standard. If you run a restaurant, spa, hotel, retail space, real estate, construction or any business, here are some realities for you to seriously consider:

Advantages of Green Practices

1. Your customers increasingly desire to do business with environment-friendly companies.
2. Many of your employees want to work for environment-friendly companies.
3. The government wants to see growth in environment-friendly companies.

4. The financial markets have begun to invest in environment-friendly companies.
5. The construction industry has environment-friendly standards to comply with.
6. More schools are demanding environment-friendly buildings.
7. New healthcare facilities are increasingly environment-friendly.
8. Individuals desire environment-friendly products and places to live, work and vacation.
9. Owners desire reductions in cost of operations and management, and an increase in employee productivity and profitability. These benefits are the result of running an environmentally-friendly business.

   No matter what kind of business you are in, I suggest that you pay close attention to the Green Movement. Stay ahead of the curve by taking steps today to go green in your business. If you do not, you will find that you will be trying to play catch-up while your competitors differentiate themselves in the marketplace. Don't be left behind!

As human beings on this planet, regardless of religion, culture, color or economic class, the gifts of this world belong to all of us. Fulfillment, happiness and nature's beauty are for all to enjoy. It is a right we earn just by being born.

ᡐ **Chapter Eight**

The Power of the Space Clearing Ritual

An unexpected part of my Feng Shui training was learning how to do a "space clearing." I had never heard of a space clearing before. When I was informed that it was a required part of the curriculum, I was taken aback. This new idea was a little too mystical for me and just the thought of it made me very uncomfortable. I was even conflicted about putting this chapter in the book. The deciding factor was looking back at the people who deeply benefited from this experience, and how it gave them a second chance in their personal lives or businesses. This chapter is not for everyone, so feel free to skip over it and move on to Chapter Nine, where I discuss how EcoChi is implemented to create wealth.

The director of the school I was attending introduced the Taoist priest who was going to spend the next four days teaching us to perform the space clearing ritual. Initially, this idea was not something I expected to ever use with my clients. I was just looking to fulfill the requirements of my studies. Much to my surprise, I found myself so fascinated by what I learned that I later went into deeper study of this ancient practice with two more esteemed teachers.

Space clearing is a method used to dissipate negative or stagnant energy (Chi). The intention of this ritual is to revitalize energy in a property while also raising the space's vibratory level. Using a variety of techniques, this ritual allows for new beginnings and sets positive intentions for the home, office or other location. Space clearings are found in most cultures and can be helpful after a stressful event, conflict, illness or death. It is also a way to change the "Predecessor Law." All of us have seen this kind of lingering bad luck. For example, a new restaurant or store opens in an old location and everyone knows that the new venture is doomed, because every business that opened there before had gone out of business. A space clearing is one of the many tools I use to remedy this situation. The clearing creates a clean palette and makes room for new energy. It is also a cathartic ceremony. My methods variously include the use of music, incense, dance, pendulum techniques, song and sound.

When performing these rituals, I work with great passion and deep intention. I understand negative energy and loss, having experienced both during challenging times in my own life. All of these events touched me in a profound way and molded me into the person I am today. I would like to share two of these experiences with you. First I will introduce you to my dear friend Goldie, whose exemplary life and courage greatly influence how I perform space clearings. I will then take you into Howard's apartment, where both of his wives died, and invite you to witness the healing powers of the space clearing ritual.

Goldie: Just Keep on Dancing

In my 15-year friendship with Goldie, she was lost to me several times. Each time, I would get a little piece of her back—only to finally lose her forever. Goldie was a little thing; even in six-inch heels she only came up to my shoulder. But she was a big presence—a bright ball of fire with a kind heart and a great passion for life. She was also meticulous about her appearance. She was always well-manicured and her thoroughly moisturized hands featured brightly colored fingertips. Her shoulder-length hair was always highlighted with blonde streaks and professionally styled. Goldie could also be recognized from a mile away because she was always resplendent in rhinestones and heart-shaped fashion pieces. Like a little magpie, she loved anything that was shiny, especially in the shape of hearts and angels!

When I met her, my husband had just moved out of our house and she had recently lost a sister to breast cancer. Both of us were devastated by our losses. We had that and so much more in common, and we became fast friends. Then, a mere three weeks after the funeral for her sister, Goldie called me at work to tell me that she had discovered a lump in her own breast. It was a cancer that she would fight for the next 15 years, until it finally won and stole her away from me, from her two teenage daughters, and from all of the other people who loved her dearly.

This was no grim friendship, but rather one of joy and laughter. Throughout her roller-coaster ride of toxic treatments and medications, we explored life together in a whole new way. We waited for the days that she felt okay, and when they came we celebrated. The Holocaust had taken all of her family except for one uncle who survived and had six children. One time between her treatments we traveled to Paris together so she could meet this uncle and the rest of her extended family. Goldie had so little family that she did not want to die without meeting these relatives. There is one image from that trip that is imbedded in my memory—Goldie dancing in the arms of her cousin, Andre, to an Andrea Bocelli aria in the living room of his home in France. He held her tightly, as if, I thought, he wanted to keep her from flying away. I did too. Andre told her in broken English how he felt; he sobbed, "I luv you Go-dee." As tears streamed down her face, she said, "I love you, too, Andre." It was the first and last time they would ever meet.

We had another adventure in Bermuda. There we searched for her housekeeper Suzanne's uncle. Suzanne had heard we were going to Bermuda for a long weekend, so she gave Goldie the name and possible location of her long-lost uncle. Goldie would not rest until we found him. She called a few phone numbers that Suzanne had given her and two days later she had tracked him down. He sent his girlfriend to pick us up from the hotel and she drove us to his house on the top of a hill. He was a Jamaican Rastafarian and beautiful to look at, a massive man with a long thick mane and smooth black skin. It was a tough neighborhood, but Goldie and I felt perfectly safe. After all, the "Rasta-Man" (as we affectionately called him) was bigger than life, and we were his guests.

During the evening, he took out a boom box and played the most enchanting reggae music I had ever heard. It was magical. As Goldie and the Rasta-Man lit up a joint (it truly was her medicine), I stepped outside. The view was breathtaking—a full moon, the sky freckled with bright stars above a lavender horizon and an azure sea. At that moment, I had a life-changing epiphany. I fully recognized that as human beings on this planet, regardless of religion, culture, color or economic class, the gifts of this world belong to all of us. Fulfillment, happiness and nature's beauty are for all to enjoy. It is a right we earn just by being born.

Deep in thought, I heard a sound, and saw that Goldie was standing beside me. "Thank you, Debbie, for taking this trip with me," she said. "You are my heart." Then she broke into a huge grin and pulled me back inside, where the music played. "Let's dance," she commanded.

Even in her darkest days, Goldie always knew there was more to life than what we see. For her, music and dance were transforming. They seemed to bring her to a place between this world and the spirit world. As the good days became increasingly rare, we embraced them with concerts and musical theater. We created moments to sing and dance whenever and wherever we could.

The last time I saw Goldie was three days before she died. She was in her bed at home, surrounded by both of her daughters. As I leaned over to talk to her she grabbed me and kissed me on my forehead, my cheeks, my eyes, my nose and mouth. I will never forget her soft little kisses and how she gently whispered, "Just keep dancing." Those very words are engraved on her headstone.

Although she did not know much about feng shui, Goldie did instinctively know that life was improved with the vibrations of music, song and dance. The more people danced in her presence, the happier she was, because it increased the positive vibrations, cleared out the old stagnant energy and opened each new day to endless possibilities. Now, whenever I perform a space clearing, I always add one or more of Goldie's transforming techniques. When I ask my clients to join me in revitalizing their spaces and their lives with sound, music, song and dance—to celebrate what was, what is and what will be—these are joyous moments in the ritual. This is no small part of Goldie's legacy, and I am grateful that you have allowed me to share her magnificent spirit with you.

Now let me take you inside a space clearing ritual.

Two Deaths in One Apartment

Howard called me in to do a space clearing after his second wife died in his New York apartment. His first wife, Nancy, had died in her sleep of a heart attack in that same apartment thirty years before. His second wife, Cheryl, was a smoker and over a two-year period died a slow death from lung cancer. She passed away in a hospital bed in the living room of this apartment. It was nine months later when we met. Understandably, Howard was having a hard time going back to the apartment after his workday. He just didn't want to be there. He thought about moving to another apartment, but the recession had hit him hard and his apartment was rent-stabilized, an asset he couldn't give up in such uncertain times.

Since there had been two deaths in the apartment, I decided to use three different space clearing techniques, layering them on top of each other. The first layer was a spiritual one. I created an altar table to honor both wives who had died in the space, and to love and nourish any energy that was not strong enough to move on to the next world. I also used a pendulum to declare the intention of this ritual, and to respectfully ask any lingering spirits for permission to clear the space. For the second layer, I used a dowsing rod to find the areas in the apartment that still held stressful energy. I also performed a practice called "smudging," using dried, smoldering herbs. I paid special attention to the areas where energies enter the space and to all other areas that were most stressed.

You can probably guess what I used for the third layer of space clearing: Goldie's technique. I brought along musical instruments, an iPod and an iPod dock to use if the opportunity for dancing presented itself.

I had prepared myself the day before by eating a vegetarian diet, meditating and taking a ritual bath with sea salt—all to neutralize my energy. The purpose of this preparation is to become a vessel, void of opinion or expectation, so that I could be totally present for the client, and for the energies I would be working with in the space.

I walked through the apartment, holding the smoking dried sage smudge stick in my hands. Following behind me, Howard said that he felt like he was going to faint. I urged him to try to hold it together. "Please do not faint," I implored. He said, "No I won't. I just feel lightheaded, like the air has changed and is lighter and clearer. It's the same feeling I get after a day of sailing, like my lungs are filled with fresh air." Clearly the space clearing had begun to work.

The Lao Pan compass is a Compass School tool that determines the magnetic direction of a space. The reading and the interpretation of the practitioner determines the best use of the different rooms. I like to call this "energy mapping" because once I have a reading I map the energies on to a floor plan. My experience shows me time and again that this is where the magic happens. This is the moment when I determine how the space is affecting a person's life.

My compass reading showed that the master bedroom in which Howard had been sleeping for over three decades was in an inauspicious area of the space. Thinking about his history in this apartment, this was no surprise. I suggested that he create a new master suite for himself in the guest room.

East has the Chi (energy) of the season of spring, and represents new beginnings. This east-facing second bedroom was full of sunshine and I was optimistic that over time this room would help him create a fresh outlook.

We also chose sunny pale yellow paint for the "Ming Tang" (entranceway).

An improved lighting design was added to create a more cheerful setting, and artwork was carefully selected to depict Howard's future aspirations. All family photographs and pictures of Cheryl were arranged with respect and dignity on a wall and altar table in the former master bedroom, which was now the guest room.

When you lose a loved one, it is difficult to remove or even *move* any of the departed's possessions, clothing, medications, even a toothbrush. Also, when someone is ready to move on to the next stages of mourning, he or she still needs lots of support. Throwing away a toothbrush sounds like an easy thing to do, but it can be a huge step for someone who is grieving. After the clearing ritual, Howard said he was ready to make these changes. He called the super in his building right away and arranged to have the apartment painted within the next two weeks. I called him to see how the painters were doing. Surprising me, he said, "My life is falling apart. When the painters started working in the old master bedroom, the entire ceiling fell down. They said nothing like this has ever happened before in this building!"

I found that very interesting. I thought for a moment and realized what had actually happened. The fallen ceiling was a physical manifestation of the space clearing. The energy from decades of illness and sorrow had literally crumbled, making way for a new ceiling and for clean, fresh energy to enter the apartment from the top down.

As of this writing, Howard is doing well. He reports that now, when he comes home, he feels like he's walking into sunshine, even during the darkest days of a New York winter. For the first time in years, he says, he's happy to be at home, uplifted by the changes we made. He is even talking about the possibility of sharing his life with someone new. His life story is ready to continue.

The work I did with Howard helped him move forward in his grieving process. His bereavement counselor recognized this, and asked me to do workshops for hospice nurses and their bereavement clients. This was an unexpected path for my business, and a most welcome opportunity to help people on their healing journey.

The Chinese have been using feng shui for thousands of years to increase prosperity and good luck in life and in business. A space clearing is one means of accomplishing this desired result, because it effectively helps to close the door on the past and make room for the future. In the next chapter I will share with you many other ways to bring in abundance. So, in honor of Goldie—and all the people in our lives, past and present, those we love and honor—play some music, sing and dance. Believe me, it will go far to raise the positive vibrations in your office, in your home, and in your heart.

I HAVE COMBINED THE BEST

ABUNDANCE TIPS FROM ALL

MY RELEVANT DISCIPLINES TO

INCREASE MY CLIENTS'

CHANCES FOR ACHIEVING

SUCCESS IN BUSINESS,

PROSPERITY AND EVEN

WEALTH.

Chapter Nine

A Home Office That Ushered In Prosperity

"How does EcoChi generate wealth?" I am asked this question over and over again by individuals, business owners and the media. The clearest way to answer this question is by relaying Kevin's story—which he has generously allowed me to share with you.

When it comes to money, we are each in different circumstances—in some cases, drastically different. Food and shelter together usually constitute our biggest expense. Add healthcare, transportation, utilities, clothing, those annual taxes that always seem to catch us by surprise, and the list can seem endless. And we haven't even gotten to such "luxuries" as televisions, computers, cell phones, life, property and auto insurance or costs for education. Add to that the fact that the post-recession economy we are living through has many of us out of work, out of money and out of luck, and you can see why money is a loaded issue for most of us, to say the least.

EcoChi is a game changer in this arena. I have combined the best abundance tips from all my relevant disciplines to increase my clients' chances for achieving business success, prosperity and even wealth. Kevin's story is a good example of how this actually works.

Kevin, Charismatic and Defeated

In his thirty years working within large companies in the New York commercial real estate business, Kevin had seen the up and down cycles that define the real estate market. When we met, the market was in the depths of a down cycle. He asked me if I would consider working with him, using my EcoChi system. We met in a coffee shop. Kevin walked in wearing a navy blue sport jacket, a light blue shirt, khaki pants and a red and blue tie. It was a cold November day and I was surprised to see that he was not wearing a coat. His hair was gray, and he had a small round bald spot on top of his head. As he approached me, I noticed deep frown lines across his forehead. We introduced ourselves and he smiled. In that warm smile, which transformed his face, I could see glimpses of his charming personality—a requisite for the successful salesman he had always been. I also saw his sincerity and integrity, reflected back at me from deep within his sky-blue eyes.

We sat in a booth and began to talk. By the time Kevin had finished two cups of half caffeinated, half decaffeinated coffee, I'd learned that his high-end sales had always been based on the close relationships he'd built over the last three decades. Now, due to the unavailability of financing and the slow-down of luxury retail sales, the real estate market was at a standstill. A divorced dad, Kevin had a mortgage to pay, hefty monthly child support payments, and for the first time in his life he had accumulated significant credit card debt. Feeling like his back was against the wall, he was willing to try any-thing. A young Korean agent in his office had told him about feng shui, and through word of mouth he found me. He was somewhat skeptical, but figured it couldn't hurt to give EcoChi, with its feng shui component, "the old college try."

To make him feel more comfortable, I shared a few unforgettable stories from my time as an active Corcoran real estate broker working with high-end residential properties, and soon enough he began telling me some of his experiences.

Finally I asked him point blank, "What do you think you should do at this point in your career?" He frowned, and the deep creases reappeared on his forehead. After a moment he replied, "Deals are so much harder to close in this environment, and here I am giving up 35% of my commission to the company I work for just to have a desk. Since all of my business comes from previous relationships, I could open my own real estate company. Doing that, even if my annual sales this year are only 65% of what they were last year, it would still be a good year for me. So that is what I probably should do." However, even as he said this he seemed hesitant, and nervously tapped his spoon on the table. In sincerity and with the hope of boosting his confidence, I agreed that it was a great strategy and reassured him that if for any reason it did not work out as expected, based on his impeccable sales history and reputation, he could always to go back to a larger company with no problem.

After this first informal meeting, we put a date on the calendar for three weeks down the road when I would visit his two-bedroom apartment on the Upper East Side of Manhattan. I also left him with my attorney's name and number so that he could pursue opening his new real estate company without delay, as I encouraged him to do. I hoped he would find the nerve to make that call and get the ball rolling.

Before I visited his residence, Kevin sent me the "EcoChi Evaluation Form" he had filled out. This form asks questions about home, career, love, work, interests, relationships, health, wants, needs, along with critical facts about birthplace and date and time of birth. I also requested a floor plan of his apartment. Within a day he e-mailed me back all of the answers plus the floor plan.

Laying out his information on my desk, I began to read the answers he provided. The questionnaire asked him to rate his life in the following areas: career, fame and wealth. He could choose a number from 1 to 10 to describe his current situation, with 1 being the lowest end of the scale. His answers looked like this: career 3, fame 3, wealth 1. These were the numbers of someone who had not closed a deal in a very long time. I could see that his confidence was broken and that I had my work cut out for me.

A Positive Discovery in Kevin's Apartment

The day arrived for my visit to Kevin's apartment. When I got there, I rolled up my sleeves and began to remove my tools from the big bag I'd brought with me. There was the Lao Pan Compass, EMF meter, measuring tape, ruler, dried herbs, Bagua (a feng shui "energy map") and musical instruments. I went outside, took a compass reading outside of his building, then came back up and took another one in the middle of his apartment to double-check the accuracy of the magnetic reading. I also calculated Kevin's "Ming Gua" (Chinese Divination) using his birthday information, noting which element was present when he took his first breath. In addition to his earth element, he was a West Life person. Each person has four lucky directions. If you are an East Life person, they are east, north, south and southeast. If you are a West Life person like Kevin, they are west, northwest, northeast and southwest. This was important information. I discovered that his direction for prosperity ("Sheng Chi") was northeast.

After drawing these energy portents onto his floor plan, I found that my initial suspicion was correct—the guest bedroom was squarely in his "Prosperity

Area." He wanted a home office, and clearly this room would be an auspicious place for him to start his new business. Further good news: Kevin told me he had already secured the certificate for the limited liability company (LLC) he needed, and that he was already working in the second bedroom!

I walked into the room to see the setup. Kevin had his desk up against the window facing out, with his back to the door. Inside my head I was screaming "No!!" In feng shui, it is very bad to have your back to a door. And having your desk line up with the entrance to the room, as Kevin's did, is even worse, because that is precisely where the Chi enters and rushes in. Energy-wise, this kind of furniture arrangement is highly unsettling. I immediately changed things around. I put Kevin into a power position by moving the desk so that his back was against the wall. In this "Black Turtle" position he could see out the window, get daylight on his desk and easily see the door to the room. Directly in front of him in his "Red Bird" position, I had him hang a framed photo of a development project he was currently pitching. Around that photo, we arranged all of the awards he had won during his highly successful career. At my request, he also had that wall painted red, a powerful color that represents the fire element, which I knew would feed his earth element. I also used low VOC paints to protect him from unnecessary airborne toxic fumes. Plants were brought in to absorb pollutants from the air and EMFs from his electronic equipment. I added tall bamboo plants to help bring in abundance. And on Kevin's desk I placed a small fish tank containing eight goldfish for good luck and one black fish to chase away any bad luck.

Chinese coins are round with a square cut out of its center. The round shape represents the Heaven Chi (energy we cannot see, including the spiritual) and the square shape represents the Earth Chi (energy of things we can see). The ancient Chinese practice of purposefully utilizing coins to attract luck and money is still used in feng shui today.

Going back to the entrance to the apartment, I tied nine lucky Chinese coins together with a red ribbon and taped them to the bottom of the welcome mat. The feng shui principle here is that as people walk into the property and step on this rug with the coins underneath, they will symbolically bring the Chi (energy) of money into the space. It is a simple but very effective use of symbolism. Next I placed the Bagua (feng shui map) over the floor plan and found that the abundance corner of the property was on the left side of the foyer. Right there we placed one of the most powerful tools for wealth—the water feature. This took the form of a beautiful Buddha fountain with water flowing up for prosperity, and a small light to enhance its power. I then placed it by a mirror to double the wealth.

The Role of the Kitchen in Attracting Wealth

People often congregate in the kitchen, but what they generally do not know is that the kitchen is a very important room for promoting wealth. In large part this comes from the fact that the better we eat the healthier we are.

A healthier person is also a more productive person who will then bring in more business. The refrigerator should be filled with healthy foods. A full refrigerator brings health, abundance and happiness. Besides the refrigerator and cabinets, I also checked the four burners on Kevin's stove, which likewise represent wealth. I told him to keep them clean and alternate his use of the burners when he cooks. He told me he did not cook, and instead ate out almost every meal, occasionally eating take-out in front of the TV.

I asked him to cook at least one meal in the apartment, once a week. I told him that even occasional cooking would turn the apartment into a home, bring more nourishment into his life, and it would be better for his health. I also recommended that he place a mirror over the stove to double the burners and thus double the wealth coming in. Lastly I did a space clearing throughout the apartment to clear out the past and make room for Kevin's new business and new life. For that I used dried sage from the Native American Oneida tribe. We meditated together and played some of the Beatles music that he loves. I also brought out a handcrafted bell and rattle to shake up the energy and we had some fun with that as well.

I could tell that Kevin was happy with what we were doing because the frown lines had disappeared from his forehead and he looked ten years younger.

Kevin, Just One Year Later...

Today Kevin is thriving as president of his own company. Although the commercial real estate market is still in a pretty deep hole, Kevin has been cashing in on his excellent reputation and longtime business relationships. For the first three quarters of 2010 he was proud to report that he had already billed $1.2 million in commissions, and he gets to keep all of it! He has now completely paid off all of his credit card debt, and as of this writing had only eight more child support payments left, since his daughter was about to graduate from George Washington University. Kevin is also well on his way to a profitable 2011 because he just signed a deal for the development that he had been pitching—yes, the exact same one displayed on his Red Bird wall. At this time Kevin was now seriously thinking of renting a new office on Madison Avenue to propel his career forward at an even faster pace. His life has taken a major positive turn on the personal front as well; he is in a committed relationship with a broker from his old office. Best of all, he has fully regained his self-confidence.

The other day Kevin called to give me an update. I had to laugh when he said, "Debra, I have to admit that I get very uncomfortable if I don't have my Buddha-Belly fountain on! The first thing I do in the morning is turn it on. I don't know why, but this really works. EcoChi has been very good to me! Can you please come to see a few offices with me before I sign a new lease?"

Wow, what a change from the downcast, depressed guy I met in the coffee shop! While I was delighted by this turn of events, none of it was surprising to me. I confess that I don't always know exactly how EcoChi creates its magic, but its power is undeniable. The results delight, amaze and nurture my clients and me every day. We did find Kevin a beautiful office, facing the northeast, and he is doing brilliantly.

Kevin's Question about Taking EcoChi on the Road

Thanks to his mushrooming business, Kevin now has meetings scheduled in China, Japan and Germany, and that is just in the next three months. He called recently to ask me what EcoChi could do for him when he travels. Specifically he wanted to know what he could do to improve his chances of walking out with the new business he was pitching—contracts signed and in his hand. So for all of you who travel for business, I would like to share the EcoChi Tips that I created to help improve Kevin's chances for success on the road.

For Business Travelers:
Increase Your Success with EcoChi

Does your hotel room truly feel like your home away from home? Follow these tips to ensure a better sleep in a healing atmosphere and put your self in a strong position for a successful outcome to your meeting.

1. **Choose your room with care.**

   • Make sure your room has windows that open, and be sure to air out the room before you go to bed.

   • Location, location, location. Choose a room that is away from vending machines, elevators, bars or restaurants, street noise and any electrical hubs such as air conditioning or heating systems.

2. **Electromagnetic Fields can interrupt a good night's sleep and affect your health.**

   • If you must keep your cell phone turned on overnight, keep it at least five feet away from you. From that distance the electromagnetic fields are much less likely to disturb you.

   • Unplug all unnecessary electronics in the room before you go to sleep, including the alarm clock next to the bed. This helps the planet by eliminating phantom energy loads, and keeps you healthier by reducing your exposure to unnecessary radio waves and EMFs. Bring a small battery alarm clock with you. For insurance, you can call the front desk and ask for a wake-up call.

3. **Small touches from home bring a sense of calm after a long day of traveling.**

   • A small travel photo frame with a picture of your love partner, friends or even your pet will bring a smile to your face and an inner feeling of peace— all necessary to allow you to be at the top of your performance. Place the frame where you can easily see it while dressing for your meeting.

• A piece of clothing that you love should be a staple in your overnight bag. It can be a beautiful scarf, tee shirt, or a ratty old hooded sweatshirt that brings you comfort. Wear it while you hang out in your room and then use it to cover the television before you go to sleep, or to cover the mirror if it is directly facing the bed. Seeing your reflection first thing when you wake up can make you uneasy and jumpy. It is important to be as calm as possible before a big meeting.

• A small scented candle is a mood-changer. Relax with your candle burning, a glass of wine or an herbal tea, and classical music–a great tool for your brain function—as you glance over the notes for your morning meeting.

4. **If you have to work in your hotel room, power up!**

• Position your chair so that your back is up against the wall and you can see the door to your room (the "Black Turtle" position in feng shui). The wall symbolically supports you and your business. The sightline to the door keeps you in power. There will be no unexpected surprises. You are in control.

• If your hotel stay is more than one night, buy a small bamboo or jade plant and place it on your desk. Bringing nature indoors makes us feel grounded. Plants naturally clean the air of toxins and absorb electromagnetic fields. These particular plants are known to bring money and success.

5. **Will they love you in the morning?**
   • Get up early enough to take a short run, walk, do yoga, qigong or tai chi, or take a short trip to the gym; 20-30 minutes is enough to get your blood circulating without draining your Chi.
   • Listen to your favorite music as you get dressed for the meeting.
   • Have breakfast. Stick to a meal that is easy to digest. If your body is working too hard, you will not be clearheaded in your meeting. Limit your caffeine intake to one or two cups maximum.
   • Choose a power position at the meeting whenever possible. The ideal is with the "Black Turtle" wall behind you, with an easy view of the door.

   Using these EcoChi strategies when you travel creates a healing atmosphere in your room and lets you get a good night's sleep. Most of all, it puts you in the position of power at meetings, increasing your odds for successful business outcomes. The money will follow. It always does. Just ask Kevin.

THE SECOND HOME IS AS

INDIVIDUAL AS THE PERSON

WHOSE HOME IT IS, BUT ITS

ROLE IS ALWAYS THE SAME:

TO HELP YOU KEEP YOUR

LIFE IN BALANCE.

The Second Home: A Special Place to Balance Your Energies

We all have the opportunity to have several homes. No, I am not talking about buying real estate. I am talking about the public spaces available to all of us. Sometimes we lose sight of the fact that there are many opportunities to find the energy and balance we need right in our own home towns and surrounding areas. The real blessing of technology is that we can do our work anywhere—on a blanket in a state park, on a seaside rock, in a library, restaurant, museum or even a sculpture garden. Every city and town has a rich plethora of environments to choose from. We are always searching for balance in our lives. This is how I found mine.

I love my city apartment in Manhattan. It is perfect for me in many ways. However, living in the heart of "the city that never sleeps" is not generally the most relaxing place to be. New York's fast-paced, vibrant, 24/7 energy is very "yang." On the positive side, it offers endless activities, opportunities and cultural events—a diverse, ever-changing smorgasbord of people, places and things. The city is a perfect arena in which to connect, build a business, keep on your game professionally and keep up with global news and views. But *whew*! Sometimes just thinking about it can exhaust me. To help keep my life in true balance, I also have a second home, one that slows me down and helps me connect and stay in tune with nature's moons, tides, rhythms and seasons.

Our yin and yang (masculine and feminine) energies are interdependent and complement each other, representing the polarities of the universe and the ever-changing balance of life. That is exactly what a second home can and should be: an opportunity to create a natural balance between these two opposite but complementary and equally necessary energies.

My second home is modest, a small ranch-style house on the North Fork of Long Island. It is situated less than half a mile from a Long Island Sound beach. To get to that stretch of beachfront, I walk on a dirt road and through an area of protected land filled with natural beauty. A full 45 acres of woods sit behind my half-acre plot of land. The house has a wonderful energy (Sheng Chi) because of its location. It is near a large body of water, and is surrounded by trees, vineyards and organic farms.

The first time I saw it, I knew that I really wanted this house. With my real estate sales down, and Manhattan showing the first signs of the soon-to-burst housing bubble, it was not however, a good time to spend that kind of money. I left a voice message for my accountant, Bob, telling him about this property I found, and how I was drawn to the place. Knowing Bob, I expected that his cooler head would prevail, and braced myself for his negative reply. When he called back, though, he delivered a mixed message that, in retrospect, was very wise.

"I understand you found an incredible deal, and that the house is priced well below others in the area," Bob said. "You also know that this is not a good time for you to do this. Financially it does not make sense, but knowing you, Debra, if you don't do it you will probably regret it for the rest of your life. You asked for my advice so here it is: Buy it, but do not renovate. Just do the minimum you need to do to get in." I was so relieved and grateful that I gushed, "I know this is very inappropriate Bob, but if you were here I would give you a great big kiss!" Through the wireless connection, I could feel him blush.

I bought the property in the spring of 2007, and I am still madly in love with it. Today I can sense and also hear the approaching end of summer. The pitter-patter of acorns as they drop on the ground is a musical sound. It reminds me of a Native American drumbeat signaling to all people, to all creatures, and to the sun and the heavens that now it is time to prepare for the new season to come. I even breathe differently in my second home. There I regain my natural rhythm. It is a source of deep happiness and celebration for me. This special place grounds me in nature and brings me closer to the elements, which I experience as a state of sheer joy. The second home is as individual as the person whose home it is, but its role is always the same—to help you keep your life in balance. We all have an innate desire to create balance in our lives. Since we are each unique, and everyone's way is somewhat different, I think it's instructive to show you how a dear friend of mine named Angelo accomplishes the feat of keeping *his* life in balance. It is quite different from my way, but the result is the same.

Angelo's Vineyards

Standing at about 5'8", Angelo is a bulky man who enjoys good food and wine. You will usually find him wearing a Yankees' cap. When he talks about his work, his whole being comes alive. His green eyes dance in his head and, in contrast to his tanned cocoa skin, they look like flashing neon lights. When he smiles and offers to shake your hand, be prepared because his hands are strong and rough with calluses. He is a true man of the earth.

Angelo's home is in Napa Valley, California, and is actually the site of his wine business. In fact, he lives in a spacious farmhouse right on his vineyard. He worked hard over many years to build his business in a way that allows it to run smoothly when he is not there. In fact, his business is now so efficiently organized and run that as soon as the grapes are harvested, Angelo hops on a plane and heads to his second home, the one-bedroom apartment he rents in the heart of Paris.

Although he loves his work and is extremely happy when he is on his vineyard, by the end of the growing season he has had far too much peace and quiet (yin energy), and he cannot wait to get back to the city that he loves and where he feels most alive. In Paris, he pursues his love of food, wine, culture and dance, and often socializes with friends well into the night. His second home in Paris provides the yang energy Angelo needs to keep his life in harmony.

Your Second Home—No Money Down, No Mortgage Needed

My story and Angelo's highlight the benefits of balancing your yin and yang energies with a second home. If you want to go out and buy a second home, all well and good, but what I am talking about here does not require the deed to an actual house!

As I suggested in the beginning of this chapter, a viable option, and one that may even be preferable, is to make an agreement with yourself that you will explore nearby neighborhoods and the outlying community until you find a public space—or several spaces—that offer you the balance you need.

Let's say you are at work, whether in an office or at home, you hit a wall and start to feel stagnant. Change your energy—and thus your mood—by heading out to a café, museum, library, park or beach. Vary your environment from time to time and I promise you that you will be pleasantly surprised at how much more can be accomplished when you return to the tasks at hand.

You can, of course, also take work with you and find renewed inspiration in a different atmosphere. In that case, pack your laptop, your papers, your notebook and a pen and head to your favorite second home—or to your favorite third or fourth home. The only limit in this case is your imagination and willingness to explore other areas both near and far.

I have included the Yin and Yang Chart to the right as a snapshot of aspects of life that offer both kinds of energy. There are times in life when movement is called for, and other times when what we need most is to be still. Over the long run, too much of either is not healthy, just as too much shade is as unhealthy as too much sun. Balance, so important to creating a healthy, happy and fulfilling life, is more readily and successfully achieved when we avoid extremes.

	YIN	YANG
Color:	black	red
Lifestyle:	too much leisure	too much hard work
Temperature:	cold	hot
Climate:	moist	dry
Weight:	heavy	light
Action:	stillness	movement
Movement:	contracting	expanding
Gender:	female	male
Energy:	negative	positive
Directions:	below	above
Architecture:	curved shape	geometrical shape
Solar Pattern:	shady area	sunny area
Numbers:	even	odd
Life Essence:	body	soul
Time of Day:	midnight	midday
Time of Year:	winter	summer

Today's children will be responsible for our planet in the years to come. With an early awakening, the right attitude and the right tools, I believe they will do a better job than we have.

❧ Chapter Eleven

The Bigger Picture:
Becoming a Global Caretaker

A dvances in technology have surpassed our dreams and expectations. Today we can shop for items from around the world in the comfort of our home and have them delivered right to our doorstep. Research to find information on virtually anything and anyone is at our fingertips. The world has shrunk. Our news is global. We carry PDAs that keep us constantly connected to each other and to the world at large. There are benefits to all of this—and major drawbacks.

I believe one challenge we face is that our plugged-in society has, to a great extent, anesthetized us to, and disconnected us from the natural world we live in. We are deafened by the cacophony of advertising and media and increasingly frustrated by political realities and unconscionable bottom-line business practices. As a result, we have lost touch with our responsibility for this planet, and all that is left is an instinctive unease concerning the depletion of its natural resources. Indeed, we have sadly forgotten how intimately and inseparably we are linked to the natural world.

One of the tenets of environmental psychology is that the healing process for our planet begins when we individually grieve for the resources we have exhausted and in some cases irreparably destroyed. When I was reading about this in my studies, it seemed like an abstract idea. Now experience has taught me that crisis is often the impetus for constructive change. In the summer of 2010, this abstract idea about grieving for the planet became personal.

A Preventable Tragedy

The BP oil spill of 2010 is an example of a devastating and, in retrospect, *preventable* turn of events that ate away at our souls. This accident severely damaged and in some cases destroyed industries, economies, marine life and our ecology. One estimate is that during this crisis between 840,000 and up to 1.7 million gallons of oil leaked into the Gulf of Mexico every single day. If this was not an assault against Mother Nature, plant life, sea life, bird life and mankind itself, then what *was* it?

Two months after the oil spill cast its dark shadow on our lives, I stood on a rocky beach on the Long Island Sound and looked out over the seemingly endless stretch of blue which defines this estuary of the Atlantic Ocean. It was a beautiful early summer day, and the clear blue water glistened in the sun. An osprey opened its massive wings above where I stood and hovered over my head as if to say hello. He was no stranger; this was the third day in a row this bird and I had met at this very same location, and the third time he welcomed me in the same way. I lifted my arms up skyward as a greeting and smiled. The sea gulls dived for shellfish and dropped their finds on the rocks, then swooped down to retrieve their succulent dinners. For the moment, all was well in my world. Such moments are precious, and they are imperative for renewing our faith in the miracle of life itself.

And then, in an instant and with no warning, it all changed. One minute I was sitting on a large rock absorbing all the beauty around me through all my senses, including my eyes, pores, lungs and heart. Suddenly, in the midst of all this beauty, I began to sob, as if I had lost a loved one. Salty tears ran down my face, and I felt a deep ache inside. I silently understood that I was grieving for what we have collectively done to damage the earth, our ecosystem and ourselves. After a while, calming myself, I released a wish to the universe that we as a species would all wake up, mourn what was done in the past, forgive ourselves and begin to rebuild our planet.

I trust that this terrible oil spill tragedy will ultimately serve as a wake-up call for others, as it did for me. It is apparent that we *are* heading in the direction of a new, far more intelligent, sensitive and constructive universal awareness.

I see it all around me; people are working hard and coming together to make things better. The fastest way to get there is one by one—each one of us waking up to the work that lies before us, which is to protect and preserve this planet we all share, for ourselves and for our children's children.

After my experience on the beach of the Long Island Sound, I made a personal commitment to create an easy-to-implement "EcoChi Sustainability Program" for my clients. I am optimistic that EcoChi will help them to rebuild our planet, one home, one office and one building at a time.

East Meets West

Eastern philosophies are based on awareness of nature as an endless cycle of transformations, rather than as a succession of unrelated phenomena. In Western culture, we name and categorize things and put them into boxes. Animals are in one box, the ocean in another, seasons in another, and human beings in yet another. This compartmentalization distances us from the reality that we are part of something much larger and grander than our daily lives. Look at the bigger picture. See the stars, the galaxies and observe how small our Earth is—a mere speck of dust in the vast horizon of space. When we accept our small part in the order of the universe, we are truly free to celebrate our place in the natural world. By shifting our perspective this way, we are able to see our planet for what it truly is, a spiritual place, our mother, our temple and our ultimate home. I believe that this is where the solution to the environmental crisis lives. When we love something this deeply we act responsibly to keep it safe—forever.

The EcoChi Circle

As an interwoven system, all three of the disciplines described earlier and briefly summarized below have been integrated into the EcoChi System. The purpose of this new design for living is to help you establish and materialize your goals, nurture your health, and bring you greater harmony and prosperity.

Classical Feng Shui is an ancient art form and system of purposefully arranging an environment so that it has a positive effect on the people who live or work there.

Green and Sustainable Living protects the environment and sustains its natural resources for today and for future generations by choosing environmentally friendly lifestyles and practices.

Environmental Psychology is an interdisciplinary science focused on the interplay between humans and their surrounding environments.

Healthy Choices is a bonus category that I added to this list, because optimal health is one of the core objectives of EcoChi.

Far eastern cultures believe that our minds, bodies and souls are intricately connected. The components of EcoChi are linked together in the same holistic manner.

Begin looking at the EcoChi diagram and you will see the concentric circles representing the components of this system. Imagine that these circles go on and on and repeat themselves into infinity. These essential disciplines interact and influence each other. They are strong enough to stand on their own, but together the whole creates an undeniable force, one that has the power to revolutionize the way we live.

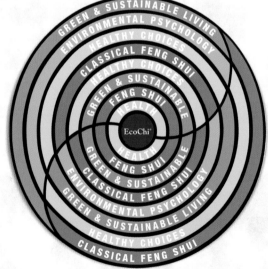

Our Hope for Our Children

Each of us as individuals has the ability to bring about change. Small steps can lead to significant change. It is my belief that the greatest impact we can have on the health of our planet is by reaching out to our children, since children learn by watching the adults in their lives. Share your commitment to the earth with your children and grandchildren. Together, make your own action plan and list what we can do to improve life on Earth. You can also bring the list below, along with your own ideas, to a local school and begin a conversation or even implement an environmental awareness program. Today's children will be responsible for our planet in the years to come. With an early awakening, the right attitude and the right tools, I believe they will do a better job than we have.

Begin Your Own Action Plan with these Ten Easy Steps

1. Volatile organic compounds are found in carpeting, paints, adhesives, finishes and fabrics. Purchase low VOC products to shield your home and office from toxins.

2. Drink filtered water instead of bottled water. All plastic bottles and containers leach chemicals into your food and drink so try to keep plastic out of your life altogether!

3. Do not run the water while you brush your teeth. Turn the faucet on only when needed. Help save our most precious resource.

4. Make conscientious purchases. Buy wooden objects and furniture made from managed forests, or buy secondhand furniture instead. Buy recycled paper products like toilet paper, paper towels and printer paper.

5. Reduce your "product carbon footprint" by purchasing locally grown produce whenever possible.

6. Bring reusable shopping bags with you to the supermarket, rather than having your groceries packed in plastic bags (plastics take 500 years to decompose).

7. Keep landfills at reasonable levels by recycling your garbage as much as possible. Paper, plastics, metals and even electronic equipment can be conveniently recycled in most towns.

8. Discontinue using toxic chemicals for lawns and property extermination. Always choose earth friendly pesticides.

9. Buy solar lights for outdoors and direct them precisely where you need the light. Do whatever you can to cut down on energy use and light pollution.

10. Set your thermostat 2 degrees higher in the summer and 2 degrees lower in the winter to cut back on energy use.

As you heal yourself, the world begins to heal.
As you heal the world, you will heal from within.

THE FUNDAMENTAL DISCIPLINES THAT MAKE UP AND SUPPORT ECOCHI—FENG SHUI, GREEN AND SUSTAINABLE PRACTICES AND ENVIRONMENTAL PSYCHOLOGY—CAN EACH, SEPARATELY AND TOGETHER, CONTRIBUTE TO ENHANCING YOUR BUILDING AND DESIGN PROJECTS, YOUR BUSINESSES, YOUR LIFE AND THE PLANET.

Chapter Twelve

A Behind-the-Curtains Look at EcoChi

At the beginning of this book, I described the life-changing day a Chinese Master told me I had a special gift that must not be wasted. From that day on, in an effort to find this gift and use it well, I have studied and learned from Chinese masters, scientists, architects, Taoist priests, shamans, professors, my clients and, continuously, from the natural world. I continue to hone my skill so that it grows and blossoms, making me even more of a finely-tuned instrument. Now, when I enter a space I can immediately feel its unique energies and those of its occupants. However, as I have discussed throughout this book, EcoChi is based on a great deal more than my intuitive abilities. In this final chapter I will explain how the fundamental disciplines that make up and support

EcoChi—feng shui, green and sustainable practices and environmental psychology—work and how they can each, separately and together, contribute to your life.

Putting the Five Elements to Work for You

The "Five Elements"—earth, metal, water, wood and fire—help us understand the movement of energy, and how they symbolize the forces within the universe. For the purpose of this book I am using the Five Elements as the building blocks to help explain the EcoChi System. I could have chosen the five senses, the organs of the human body, or the seasons of the year, because EcoChi is directly intertwined with all the patterns and cycles of life. My objective in choosing the Five Elements is to make these teachings as user-friendly as possible.

For each element I have listed feng shui, green and sustainable living and environmental psychology tips and suggestions for your work and living spaces. The EcoChi System also focuses on healthy choices for individuals, businesses and the planet. EcoChi has the ability to improve our buildings, our businesses and our lives when put into action. It is the *combination* of the disciplines that catalyzes its power. The suggestions below are easy to implement and will allow you to make informed choices that positively influence your happiness, prosperity, health and well-being.

Keep in mind that this formula is not fixed and static but rather fluid and evolving. I regularly adapt my methods with additional strategies from such cutting edge disciplines as sacred geometry, biomimicry, Bau-biologie, along with new discoveries and revelations gleaned from modern scientists and health gurus. In other words, EcoChi is as alive, dynamic and as evolving as life itself.

THE FIRE ELEMENT

In Feng Shui, yang or *male energy* rooms (as opposed to yin, or female energy) are the active rooms. These will benefit from the fire energy of the sun. Before construction, floor plans should be created to insure that the sun will shine in the yang rooms of a space—living room, playroom, kitchen and offices. If a yang room must be in a dark (yin) area of the property, I suggest painting one wall red or adding red or orange decorative accessories to bring in the fire element.

Green and Sustainable Living – As a LEED® Professional I always ask, "Where is the sun in respect to your property?" When designing a residential or commercial building, consider maximizing the sun's ability to warm it in the winter and with strategic landscaping, keep it cool in the summer. One way to accomplish this is by planting trees that are in full bloom and produce shade in the summer and lose their leaves in winter, letting more sun in when the sun is most needed to warm the property.

Additional suggestions for utilizing the sun or the fire element are:

1. Use solar shades to control the heat and glare in your space. The sun is a light source that is always on the move. Proper window coverings give you the power to manipulate daylight for your individual needs.

2. Consider solar panels as an energy source. Talk to your contractor about tax advantages and rebates for converting to onsite solar energy. If this is not practical, inquire about purchasing Green Power from your energy provider. Prices may be up to 15% more for Green Power in some areas, but these prices are coming down quickly and there are programs with long-term savings and other advantages.

3. Update your lighting to include compact florescent light bulbs. Just changing the six incandescent bulbs you use most often will save over $100 a year on your energy bills.

Environmental Psychology – Environmental Psychology tells us that not only is sunlight of great importance to the normal functioning of all living creatures and plants, but also that it makes us healthier, happier and more productive. With this in mind, consider full-spectrum light bulbs when shopping for lighting. They closely resemble natural daylight, create a vibrant, white light and elevate moods.

Healthy Choices – Light pollution is a common problem, one caused by a design flaw in most lighting design and lamps. Too often, light is allowed to shine up and out into the sky, instead of focusing light right down here, where we need it. Most life forms depend on dark nights to stay in a natural rhythm. Sadly, today our bodies are being fooled by 24 hours of daytime because of light pollution in our homes and on our city streets. This can make it challenging to get a good night's sleep. Keep blackout shades in your bedroom, only use outdoor lighting when needed and *point those lights down!*

THE EARTH ELEMENT

In Feng Shui, heavy objects represent earth energy. The dining room is a good place to have heavy furniture. It is believed that the energy of weighty chairs and tables will aid digestion.

Green and Sustainable Living The earth is what grounds us. It also nourishes and supports us. It is what we stand on—flooring, outdoor spaces, grass and soil. Here are some things you can do to honor the earth element:

1. Soil from potted plants helps to balance and absorb toxins from the indoor environment. Grow food and herbs in organic soil near your window. They smell great, taste good and nourish you!

2. Heat your building from the earth up. Geothermal heating systems harness the earth's heat from 15 feet below the surface. Traditional water-based

heating systems require twice as much electricity as geothermal systems.
3. Concrete countertops are very much in style and can be environmentally friendly. Do shop carefully for concrete countertops and ask questions. Some concrete mixtures are "greener" than others. Ask the contractor for a product that includes the use of recycled waste materials in the mix.

Environmental Psychology — We all have times when our lives seem out of control, and we need to ground ourselves. In those times, head outdoors! Plant your feet on the ground and raise your arms to the heavens. Take deep breaths. Consciously breathe in and out. You may even want to find a big old wise tree. Sit under it, put your hand on the trunk, smooth its leaves, feel its sturdiness and wisdom. Gardening has the same effect. Put your naked hands deep into the soil. It will make you feel closer to Mother Earth.

Healthy Choices — Have your building or home checked for radon. Radon is an odorless, tasteless and colorless cancer-causing gas. It is naturally created by the radioactive breakdown of uranium in the soil, rocks and moisture in the earth. If you find radon in your building, a professional can create a venting system that will draw the radon from the bottom of the home through pipes and eliminate the fumes by passing them out through the roof.

THE METAL ELEMENT

Feng Shui —This ancient art informs us that metal wind chimes can be hung in any area that encounters stagnant Chi. It is most effective near a doorway or window. The movement of the door or the wind will create a vibration and the chimes will ring. Be sure to choose the sound of your chimes carefully. It should be pleasant and calming.

Green and Sustainable Living — Our buildings get their strength from metal. A much-needed resource, metal is used to create sturdy structures, wiring, technology and appliances. Show your respect for the metal element with these practices:

1. Recycle metals! Metals are valuable and are the perfect candidates for "upcycling." This is a process that brings sustainability to a new level. Upcycling takes place when waste materials are used to manufacture new merchandise that is sometimes even more valuable than the original product. If you have a large quantity of waste metal, you can sell it. Research resources in your area to find potential buyers.

2. Don't blow a fuse! Update all electrical wiring. More efficient wiring saves you unnecessary overload, and getting rid of mazes of worn wires is an easy way to prevent an electrical fire.

3. Unplug appliances! Even when your appliances are turned off, if they are plugged into the outlets you still are being charged for electricity.

Environmental Psychology — Designing with metal sculptures, coins or rich metallic fabrics creates a feeling of opulence. If you see wealth represented in your environment you feel affluent. Feeling abundance brings more abundance because you are more likely to be making confident decisions.

Healthy Choices — Metals conduct electric magnetic fields from nearby electronics and can lead to disturbed sleep and other health problems. Try as much as possible to keep metals out of your bedroom. A metal headboard and metal spring mattress may be the cause of your insomnia.

THE WATER ELEMENT

Feng Shui — Water is the element most closely linked to prosperity. To keep wealth from flowing out, make sure you have no leaks in your plumbing and that your toilet seats are in the down position when not in use. Place a water feature, such as a fountain or a miniature waterfall, in the southwest corner of your property and watch greater abundance enter your life. Remember to always keep the water and the fountain itself clean.

Green and Sustainable Living — Did you know why it feels wonderful to be near a large body of water? This is because our bodies are 70% water. The movement of the water calms and heals us. Water is also a precious resource.

Consider this: 98% of the water on our planet is saltwater, and is therefore unusable. With so little usable water, are you doing your part to ensure our water supply for the future? Here are some suggestions:

1. Replace old toilets with low flush toilets. For approximately $300, you can purchase a new 1.6 gallon per flush toilet that will pay for itself in six years and will save over 180,000 gallons of water in that six-year period.

2. Do not prewash your dishes before putting them in your dishwasher. Dishwashers today are made to do the whole job. You save more water by using the dishwasher than by hand-washing your dishes. If you must pre-wash, use a tub in the sink so that you are reusing the water instead of letting the water run.

3. Save lots of water through thoughtful landscaping. For example, use native plantings that require little or no watering.

Environmental Psychology — Whether it is natural or man-made, people love to be near water. They gather around fountains all over the world. The sound comforts us, the splashing delights us. Hours can go by as we entertain ourselves by peering into a small fish tank or an aquarium. It makes us happy. We are reminded that we are a small part of something grand.

Healthy Choices — Drink filtered water instead of bottled water, and ideally use a non-plastic, reusable container. Hundreds of miles out at sea, if you skim the top of the water with a net, what do you think you find? Plastic! It takes over

500 years for a piece of plastic to decompose and plastic is everywhere. Piles of plastic are growing at an alarming rate. The secret chemicals that create plastic products are found in our food and our landfills. When recycled, they release toxins into the air. Rethink your purchase of bottled water.

THE WOOD ELEMENT

Feng Shui — The wood energy symbolizes rebirth and growth and is represented by the color green. Place a small tree in your office or even a picture of trees to promote the growth of your career or business.

Green and Sustainable Living — How many buildings have you seen that were constructed without the use of wood? Few indeed! As a species we love wood. Wood is strong; it breathes, aids in ventilation, absorbs sounds, is warm to the touch and is available in a large variety of textures and colors. It is nature's art. Sadly, however, we have been abusing our trees and forests for decades. You can help by keeping these things in mind:

1. Save our precious resources by buying wood that comes from managed forests. One example is the Forest Stewardship Council. The FSC is a not-for-profit organization established to promote responsible management of the world's forests.
2. Select your new wood from sustainable trees such as cedar, Douglas fir

and pine trees. Another wonderful option is bamboo, which is a rapidly renewable resource that is not classified as a tree, because it is actually a fast-growing grass.

3. Help cut down on carbon emissions created by the transporting of goods. Buy furniture and wood supplies locally. Secondhand or recycled furniture is also a great option.

Environmental Psychology — The rich green of an emerald is one of nature's most beautiful sculptures. In its most valuable form, it comes close to the color of grass and the lotus leaf. These are the colors of wood energy. Decorating with this color stimulates new ideas and expands the creative mind. It is the color of new beginnings.

Healthy Choices – Wood is one of the healthiest building materials. Be sure that all varnishes and stains have low or no VOCs. People with allergies may need to completely avoid pine resins.

THE AIR ELEMENT

Bonus (The "Feng" of Feng Shui means wind)

Feng Shui – What is the natural air flow in your space, and how does the Chi flow? If energy is stagnant, refresh it with a ceiling fan, wind chimes, incense or the good vibrations of music. For tough jobs, a professional space clearing is sure to be uplifting, and will give you a fresh perspective.

Green and Sustainable Living — If there is no fresh air in a space, then the space changes quickly. Any imbalance triggers an effort by the forces of nature to seek correction. In this effort to regain balance, growths will then be produced rapidly, leading to what can become serious mold, mildew and dust mite problems. Following are some ways you can improve the air element around you:

1. Give your space an air bath! For natural ventilation, turn off the air conditioning unit and open the windows. The benefit to the environment is a reduction in energy use and a reduction in the levels of ozone depletion caused by the use of refrigerants. Another added plus is the reduction you will see in your energy bills.

2. Bring nature indoors. Plants clean the air. They have tiny pores in their leaves that act as air filters. It is through these tiny holes that they remove toxins from the atmosphere. NASA studies show that "golden pothos" are the most effective indoor plants for removing formaldehyde molecules. Flowering plants such as gerbera daisy and chrysanthemums remove benzene from the air. Other good performers are *Dracaena Massangeana* and *Spathiphyllum*.

3. Plug up any air leaks around windows, doorways and ductwork. This is an easy way to reduce energy use by up to 20%. It is so simple that you can do it yourself in one weekend with a tube of caulk.

Environmental Psychology – Shield the front door of your home from the effects of a cold winter wind with a thoughtful landscaping design. Keep in mind that secluded entrances can create a feeling of vulnerability. Install an outdoor light with a motion detector. This is a good security precaution that creates a feeling of control and empowerment.

Healthy Choices – There are more than 75,000 synthetic volatile organic compounds (VOCs) in our building materials and furnishings. These extremely harmful toxins are inside our homes and buildings, and are being released or off-gassed into the air we breathe. Be aware of the materials you use and how they are installed. Choose low VOC paints and finishes, and natural materials for carpeting and fabrics.

A Final Word

I hope you have enjoyed learning about EcoChi and the elements that went into its creation. My intention is that you are left with a fresh perspective on your projects, your businesses, your life and the "life" of your spaces. My hope is that you utilize this book as a reference guide and that it helps you to make some productive and enriching changes in your own environments. I have included a glossary and an index at the end of the book so you can easily review areas of interest. I would also like to invite you to visit www.LivingHomeBy-

Debra.com and www.ecochi.com. These websites have a wealth of content that may prove helpful, including links to my blog, videos, social networking sites and other resources. I hope you will also sign up for my newsletter, The EcoChi News, for updates as I continue to share my journey with you.

What I have learned so far on my path, through the roller coaster of personal challenges, the intensive studies, my clients' transformations and ultimately the creation of EcoChi is this: Each of us is both a part of—and a perfect replica of—the unending, interconnected web of life. This is the universal energy from which we come and to which we return. That is why, when our spaces are thoughtfully designed to align with the natural world, they support and nourish us in unimaginable ways and, in so doing, allow us to live infinitely healthier and happier lives.

This is my heartfelt aspiration for you…Namaste.

"Become totally empty.
Let your heart be at peace.
Amidst the rush of worldly comings and goings
Observe how endings become beginnings..."

~from the Tao Te Ching by Lao-Tzu

Glossary of Terms

The 5 Elements: earth, metal, water, wood, fire.

Earth: This element's season is late summer. Its energy moves horizontally, and like the soil, it is in a stage of gathering in a downward and inward motion. Earth's energy is balanced, centered and grounded. The shape associated with Earth is flat or square. The color representing Earth is yellow.

Metal: The season that represents Metal energy is autumn. This energy symbolizes work well done and time to contract by moving within and becoming still. Metal energy is precise and logical. Round and dome-like shapes are characteristic of the Metal element. The colors associated with Metal are white, gray, silver and light pastels.

Water: Winter is the season of Water. It is wavy, deep moving energy. Water portrays a depth of emotion and introspection. It suggests the inner self, the beginning of a more relaxed, more flexible stage. The shape of Water is uneven and irregular. The colors associated with the Water element are black and dark blue.

Wood: Representing rebirth, the Wood element is the season of spring. Wood energy is an upward, expansive movement and symbolizes growth. It is influential and flexible. It is an "awakening" bursting with new vitality. The shape of the Wood element is a rectangle. The color is green.

Fire: Summer is the season of Fire. This element can bring warmth, light and heat but can also explode like a volcano. Fire energy is very active and vibrant. It is energy with an outward and expanding movement. It is triangular in shape and is represented by the color red.

Feng Shui Definitions, A through Z

Auspicious: Often used in feng shui and astrology to denote positive influences and favorable conditions. The term connotes beneficial effects and successful results or good luck.

Bagua: The Bagua is considered the map of feng shui. The energy of the rising sun is in the East, the warmest sun high in the South, setting sun in the West, and the energy of night below in the North. The Bagua charts the cyclical energies of the universe and is a valuable tool in all schools of feng shui.

Bazhai: Ba means 8 and zhai means house in Chinese. Bazhai is the most popular method of Classical Feng Shui, which is also known as Compass School. The influences of the Chi of a property are studied to see if the space's layout is in harmony with the person living or working in that space.

Black Turtle (Tortoise): This dark, hard-shelled warrior symbolizes support and protects our back from wind, enemies and unexpected inauspicious energy. Outdoors it refers to mountains, hills, trees, buildings or fences. Indoors, a wall, screen or plant is used as a Black Turtle. You are in a power position when it is behind your bed and desk.

Chi (Qi, Ki): Chi blankets the entire universe. Scientifically speaking, it is the intelligence-holding vibration of subatomic particles that make up all matter. In the United States, the description most closely aligned with this concept is "life force." Chi is most often invisible and is made up of Sheng Chi and Sha Chi. Sheng Chi moves in waves and curves and is the Chi of natural formations. Sha Chi is found in and around man-made shapes and often travels in straight lines. Feng shui brings harmony by maximizing and containing the Sheng Chi and reducing the Sha Chi. This balance encourages health, happiness and prosperity.

Clutter: Too many items in a space will obstruct the Chi. Clutter can be physical, emotional or spiritual and creates negative or stagnant energy.

Electromagnetic Fields (EMFs): These are magnetic energy fields. Wherever there is electric current, there are EMFs. Over-exposure to electromagnetic fields is believed to be harmful to our health.

Feng Shui: In Cantonese Feng Shui (Fung Shway) literally means "wind and water." These are the forces that shape our environment. One is visible (water) and the other invisible (wind). In the broad view, it stands for the relationship between surrounding nature, landscape, the beauty of buildings and the happiness of the inhabitants. It is a system of purposefully arranging an environment so that it has a positive effect on the people who live, work or visit there.

I Ching: It is an ancient philosophical text known as "The Book of Changes." It has the oldest descriptions and observations of nature. The I Ching has been used to guide and protect people for thousands of years.

Inauspicious: This word is frequently used in feng shui and astrology. It describes undesirable or harmful influences. It is also used to denote unfavorable, unsuccessful results or being unlucky.

Lo Shu Square (Magic Square): It is a mathematical grid used in feng shui numerology. Myth tells us that the numbers were discovered on the shell of a giant turtle. It is a 3x3 grid called a magic square, because any three numbers in a line add up to 15.

Lao Pan Compass: This is a tool used by those in the Compass School to determine best directions and solar orientation for a building. It measures magnetic directions and has a complex system of rings that reveal feng shui information.

Namaste: Means, "I honor the Spirit in you, which is also in me." This globally popular salutation is used when either greeting or leaving someone you like and respect. It is believed to have originated in India and Nepal.

Poison Arrow (Cutting Chi): Poison arrows are sharp angular lines directed towards you. Jagged edges of buildings directed towards the home, table corners, straight roads and pointed objects are all examples of poison arrows. It is an inauspicious energy.

Red Bird (Phoenix): The Red Bird is in front of you. In Compass School it is the Facing or Water direction. Indoors, it is the direction you face when sitting. In feng shui it can be a powerful tool that can be used to shape your future.

San Cai: The San Cai is known as the Three Gifts of Heaven, Earth and Humanity. An essential principle of feng shui and Taoist teachings, these three energies in balance lead to good fortune and health.

Space Clearing: A method used to dissipate negative or stagnant energy (Chi), Space clearing rituals raise the vibratory level and revitalize spaces. By using a variety of techniques and creating a clean palate, it allows for new beginnings and setting intentions. Space clearing is found in most cultures and can be helpful after a stressful event, conflict, illness or death. It is also a wonderful ceremony to cleanse the energy of a property before moving in, to make way for a new life. Methods can include the use of music, incense, pendulum techniques, dance and sound.

Yin and Yang: It is believed that the complimentary energies of yin and yang represent the ever changing balance of life and the universe. Yang represents masculine, active, rigid and strong energy. Yin symbolizes darkness, stillness, weakness and the feminine energy.

Green Definitions

Acid Rain: The term acid rain describes the several ways that acidic compounds fall out of the atmosphere and cause a variety of ground-level environmental effects. These effects compromise human health and include damage to forests and soils, fish and other living things.

Adapted plants: These are low maintenance plants that are not native to a habitat. The plants are hardy, noninvasive, and need little protection, pest control, fertilization or watering.

Brownfield: A site that was previously used for commercial or industrial purposes that is contaminated with toxins or pollutants. It has the potential to be reused once it is cleaned up.

Carbon Footprint: A measure of greenhouse gases that estimate how much carbon dioxide an entity or product produces and releases into the atmosphere.

Climate Change: Significant changes in climate caused by nature or by human activities that modify the atmosphere's established order.

Coal: A fossil fuel that is a dark brown or black solid. It is naturally formed from fossilized plants and animal matter that has been subjected to geologic heat and pressure over millions of years. It is a readily available resource in the United States and provides about half of the nation's electricity. However, coal-fired power plants generally cause more pollution per unit of electricity than any other fuel. The proposed development of so-called "clean coal" is highly controversial, as some parties believe no such development is possible and that it is misleading and a contradiction in terms.

Energy Efficiency: Energy efficiency refers to products or systems using less energy to do the same or better job than conventional products or systems. Energy efficiency saves energy, saves money on utility bills, and helps protect the environment by reducing the amount of electricity that needs to be generated.

When buying or replacing products or appliances for your home, look for the ENERGY STAR® label (EPA)

Energy Star: A federal program that labels household products that have met energy-efficient standards set by the U.S. Environmental Protection Agency and the U.S. Department of Energy. They also have a widely used energy rating system for buildings.

Go Green: To "Go Green" is to participate in environmentally friendly lifestyles and choices. The intention is to create ecological integrity by helping to protect the environment and sustain its natural resources.

Green Power: Electricity that is generated from renewable energy sources is often referred to as "green power." Green power products can include electricity generated exclusively from renewable resources or, more frequently, electricity produced from a combination of fossil and renewable resources. Also known as "blended" products, these typically have lower prices than 100 percent renewable products. (EPA)

Greenwashing: Greenwashing is a deceptive use of "green PR" or "green marketing." It is the practice of some companies to disingenuously spin their products and policies as environmentally friendly.

LEED®: Stands for "Leadership in Energy and Environmental Design." It is a Green Building Rating System and independent certification program that provides voluntary guidelines for developing energy efficient, sustainable buildings. Created by the U.S. Green Building Council, LEED® concentrates its efforts on improving performance across five key areas: energy efficiency, indoor environmental quality, materials and resources, sustainable site development and water quality and efficiency.

Native plants: Growing in a particular area before humans introduced plants from distant places, these plants are vigorous and hardy, and they are resistant to most pests and diseases. This kind of landscaping takes little maintenance and requires no irrigation or fertilization.

Off-gassing: The process by which volatile compounds evaporate and release chemicals into the air. Materials such as paints, varnishes, carpet, flooring, insulation, countertops, kitchen cabinets, plywood or particleboard, paint strippers and furniture can produce significant off-gassing. Fumes from volatile organic compounds (VOCs) affect the quality of indoor air and can create serious health problems.

Renewable Energy: The term renewable energy generally refers to electricity supplied from renewable energy sources, such as wind and solar power, geothermal, hydropower, and various forms of biomass. These energy sources are considered renewable sources because they are continuously replenished on the Earth. (EPA)

Smog: Smog is the brownish haze that pollutes our air, particularly over cities in the summertime. Smog can make it difficult for some people to breathe and greatly reduces how far we can see through the air. The primary component of smog is ozone, a gas that is created when nitrogen oxides react with other chemicals in the atmosphere, especially in strong sunlight. (EPA)

Sustainability: The traditional definition of sustainability calls for policies and strategies that meet society's present needs without compromising the ability of future generations to meet their own needs. (EPA)

Rapidly Renewable Materials: Resources that can be rapidly replenished as they are being used. Some woods, grasses, cork and bamboo replenish faster than hardwoods, and fall into the category that is considered rapidly renewable materials.

VOCs: Volatile organic compounds are gasses emitted and released into the air by a wide range of products. Examples include but are not limited to paints and lacquers, cleaning supplies, pesticides, building materials, furnishings, copiers and printers, permanent markers, craft materials including glues and adhesives, and photographic chemicals. Pollution that is indoors can be up to five times worse than outdoor pollution, due to high levels of VOCs.

Definitions of Emerging Disciplines

Bau-biologie: This practice, which originated in Germany, takes the conditions found in natural environments and brings them into the home environment. Bau-biologie, literally translated from the German, is "building biology." It creates a holistic interaction between man-made structures and the health of all life and living environments. The intention is that this natural environment will contribute to the occupant's health of body, mind and spirit, and at the same time have a low impact on the ecosystem.

Bio-Architecture: This is the study of the natural principles of animal and human-made structures. It is an organic architecture that offers a design approach arising from natural principles, and gives us buildings that are in harmony with nature.

Biomimicry: This new term comes from "bios" which means life, and "mimesis," which means to imitate. It is an emerging discipline that studies nature's best ideas and then imitates these processes and designs in an attempt to help solve the challenges and problems of the human species.

EcoChi ~ Designing the Human Experience

*EcoChi: A new design concept, developed by Debra Duneier, that blends Classical Feng Shui, Green and Sustainable Living, Environmental Psychology and a variety of emerging disciplines, to revolutionize how people feel in their space. By bringing nature's elements indoors in a whole new way, the EcoChi system attracts prosperity, harmony, health, happiness and environmental integrity.

Environmental Psychology: An interdisciplinary science focused on the interplay between humans and their surrounding environments. The field defines the term broadly, including natural environments, built environments, learning, social, and informational environments. It is believed that protecting, rebuilding and creating a preferred environment, increases the sense of well-being and behavioral effectiveness in humans.

Sacred Geometry: The use of a select group of mathematical ratios to create forms. Imagine life from seed to flower, flower to fruit, fruit to seed—re-creating and re-creating. That is one of many examples of sacred geometry in its natural state. Some architects and designers may draw upon the concept of sacred geometry when they choose specific geometric forms to intentionally create harmonic, calming, spiritual and soul-satisfying spaces.

Index

Index

Index

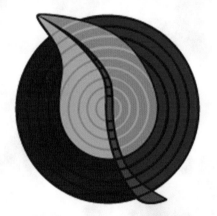

EcoChi®

EcoChi is a registered trademark